INTERMITTENT FASTING FOR WOMEN

How to Build a Personalized Routine for Weight Loss and Reverse the Signs of Aging through the Keto Meal and Exercise Plan

By

Sasha Taylor

TABLE OF CONTENTS

CHAPTER ONE

INTERMITTENT FASTING

INTRODUCTION

Intermittent fasting (IF) is presently one of the world's most popular wellbeing and wellness patterns. Individuals are utilizing it to get in shape, improve their wellbeing and streamline their ways of life.

Numerous investigations show that it can affect your body and mind and may even assist you with living longer. Intermittent fasting may somewhat support digestion while helping you eat less calories. It's a compelling method to get more fit and reduce fat.

Three nourishing meals daily is the standard in the world, yet as far as human advancement, it's a generally new thought. The breakfast-lunch-meal routine was likely settled by Europeans, some of whom laughed at the "boorish" Native Americans who didn't have unbending eating times and changed dietary propensities with the seasons. Be that as it may, as Yale University educator and creator of *Food: The History of Taste*, Paul Freedman, contends, there's no natural purpose behind eating three meals every day at explicit occasions.

Research shows that supplanting repetitive dietary patterns with controlled fasting can be helpful for your wellbeing, especially through intermittent fasting, which can include fasting for a few days one after another, fasting for 18 hours every day and eating just during the remaining six, and comparable methodologies.

Intermittent fasting is by all accounts the new pattern twirling among society. Intermittent fasting is a foreordained period in which an individual intentionally doesn't eat. There are a wide range of fasting strategies, much the same as there are numerous sorts of diets. From the 12-hour fast to the other day fasting, there are numerous sorts of fasts that are getting progressively famous. The idea behind intermittent fasting is that after the body is drained of sugars, it begins to consume fat around 12-24 hours after starvation so subsequently keeping the body from food for 12-24 hours will conceivably prompt weight reduction which can improve wellbeing. Be that as it may, the vast majority of the investigations done on this subject have been performed on animals over a brief period and have estimated glucose levels instead of long-haul wellbeing results. Many contend that intermittent fasting isn't really perilous, yet numerous additionally concur that intermittent fasting isn't all right for everybody. So truly, it is conceivable to lose calories, fat and weight from this mainstream diet, but it is likewise conceivable to, similarly as fast, restore the weight, grow low vitality stores which can bring about a discouraged state of mind, issues with dozing and even organ harm if the fasting is outrageous. Coming up next are reasons why people ought to stay away from intermittent fasting:

You ought to abstain from fasting inside and out if that you have higher caloric needs:

People who are underweight, battling with weight increase, under 18 years old, pregnant or who are breastfeeding should not attempt an intermittent fasting diet, as they need adequate calories every day for legitimate advancement.

You ought to abstain from fasting if that you are in danger of a dietary problem:

Intermittent fasting has a high relationship with bulimia nervosa, and therefore, people who are vulnerable to a dietary problem ought not to experience any eating routine related with fasting. Hazard factors for a dietary problem include having a relative with a dietary problem, compulsiveness, impulsivity and state of mind shakiness.

You will in all probability feel hungry, gorge, become dried out, feel tired and be bad tempered.

Intermittent fasting isn't for the weak-willed, implying that regardless of whether you are not underweight, you are more than 18 years old, you are not inclined to a dietary problem, and you are not pregnant or breastfeeding, you will undoubtedly have some undesirable symptoms.

Without a doubt, you will see your stomach protesting during fasting periods, basically if that you are used to consistent brushing for the duration of the day. To maintain a strategic distance from these appetite torments during fasting periods, abstain from taking a gander at, smelling, or in any event, considering food, which can trigger the arrival of gastric corrosive into your stomach and cause you to feel hungry.

Non-fasting days are not days when you can go overboard on anything you desire as this can prompt weight gain. Fasting may likewise prompt an expansion in the pressure hormone, cortisol, which may prompt much more food longings. Remember that indulging and voraciously consuming food are two basic symptoms of intermittent fasting.

To expose this fantasy effectively, intermittent fasting isn't really an eating routine, since it doesn't confine you from eating a specific food. In principle, you can have an eating routine comprising of just pizza and brew, and you will get in shape as long as you keep up a caloric deficiency.

Obviously, this isn't prudent, as in spite of the fact that you will get thinner, you won't be anyplace close to sound with that sort of utilization. Despite everything, it's better to adhere to a decent eating routine comprising of entire foods plentiful in protein, fiber, and nutrients. You can have a slice of pizza now and then, however, don't make it your staple.

Intermittent fasting is only a guide on when you ought to eat, and when you ought not to eat. It's anything but a prevailing fashion or crash diet that guarantees mysterious body changes if that you restrict yourself from certain foods.

CHAPTER TWO

WHAT IS INTERMITTENT FASTING?

Intermittent fasting (IF) is an eating design that cycles between times of fasting and eating. It doesn't determine which foods you ought to eat but instead when you ought to eat them. Right now, it is not an eating routine in the customary sense but rather, more precisely portrayed as an eating design.

Basic intermittent fasting techniques include every day 16-hour fasts or fasting for 24 hours, two times every week.

Fasting has been a training all through human development. Hunter gatherers didn't have general stores, coolers or food accessible all year. In some cases, they couldn't find anything to eat.

Thus, people advanced to survive without food for expanded timeframes. Truth be told, fasting now and again is more normal than continually eating 3–4 (or more) meals every day. Fasting is additionally regularly accomplished for strict or profound reasons, such as in Islam, Christianity, Judaism and Buddhism.

Intermittent fasting is designed around a simpler

model and good old-fashioned calorie constraint. "Intermittent fasting can be achieved in a number of ways. The overall basis, though, is based on a period of extensive time where you go without eating—which is the fast. Many people on IF regime do this for 12-16 hours all night, and eat their first food at lunch or mid-morning." Not only are calories reduced this way, but IF lovers also believe the timetable helps with digestion as well. In addition, IF seems to be highly valuable: a recent summary of research on intermittent fasting found that, if you're in excellent physical and emotional fitness, this kind of plan on its own won't affect you. Certainly, almost any intermittent fasting plan is going to end in some level of weight loss, too, according to the overview's authors of the resent research on IF.

CHAPTER THREE

BENEFITS AND DISADVANTAGES OF

INTERMITTENT FASTING

Benefits of fasting

Mental balance: It has been medically proven by psychiatrists that periodic fasting can improve human cognitive function. All the food we ingest go through the gut, and abstinence from meals helps the gut to do less work.

It reduces the rate of inflammation and stress: Oxidative stress is always reduced when you fast; it also reduces insulin resistance and aids in the reduction of inflammation.

Here are the principle medical advantages of intermittent fasting:

Weight reduction: As referenced above, intermittent fasting can assist you with shedding pounds and paunch fat, without having to deliberately limit calories.

Insulin obstruction: Intermittent fasting can decrease

insulin opposition, bringing down glucose by 3–6% and insulin levels by 20–31%, which ought to ensure against type 2 diabetes.

Aggravation: Some investigations show decreases in markers of irritation, a key driver of numerous ceaseless ailments.

Heart wellbeing: Intermittent fasting may diminish "terrible" LDL cholesterol, blood triglycerides, incendiary markers, glucose and insulin opposition— all hazard factors for coronary illness.

Disease: Animal investigations recommend that intermittent fasting may prevent malignant growth.

Mind wellbeing: Intermittent fasting expands the cerebrum hormone BDNF and may help the development of new nerve cells. It might likewise secure against Alzheimer's infection.

Against maturing: Intermittent fasting can expand life expectancy in rodents. Studies indicated that fasted rodents lived 36–83% longer.

Remember that examination is still in its beginning periods. A significant number of the examinations were little, present moment or directed in animals. Numerous inquiries still can't seem to be replied in greater human investigations.

Rundown

Intermittent fasting can have numerous advantages for your body and cerebrum. It can cause weight reduction and may decrease your danger of type 2 diabetes, coronary illness and malignant growth. It might likewise assist you with living longer.

Makes Your Healthy Lifestyle Simpler

Eating well is straightforward, however it tends to be unimaginably difficult to keep up. One of the principle deterrents is all the work required to anticipate and prepare sound meals.

Intermittent fasting can make things simpler, as you don't have to plan, concoct or clean after the same number of meals as in the past. Therefore, intermittent fasting is extremely mainstream among the life-hacking swarm, as it improves your wellbeing while simultaneously rearranging your life.

One of the significant advantages of intermittent fasting is that it makes smart dieting less difficult. There are less meals you have to get ready, concoct and clean after.

Intermittent fasting benefits

Intermittent fasting's most evident advantage is weight loss. However, there are numerous potential advantages past this, some of which have been known since the olden days.

The fasting time frames were frequently called 'washes down', 'detoxifications', or 'refinements', yet the thought is comparative—for example, to go without eating food for a specific timeframe, regularly for wellbeing reasons. Individuals envisioned that this time of forbearance from food would free their bodies' frameworks from poisons and restore them. They may have been more right than they knew.

More advantages of intermittent fasting include:

- Aids in fat burning
- Brings down blood insulin and sugar levels
- Improved mental lucidity and concentration
- Improved blood cholesterol profile
- Conceivably longer life
- Actuation of cell purifying by invigorating autophagy
- Decrease of inflammation

Also, fasting offers numerous significant, exceptional and favorable circumstances that are not accessible in average weight control plans.

Where diets can entangle life, intermittent fasting may disentangle it. Where diets can be costly, intermittent fasting can be free. Where diets can require significant investment, fasting spares time. Where diets might be restricted in their accessibility, fasting is accessible anyplace. Also, as aforementioned, fasting is an amazing strategy for bringing down insulin and diminishing body weight.

Intermittent fasting helps in weight reduction

Adjusting eating and fasting

At its very center, intermittent fasting basically permits the body to utilize its put-away vitality. For instance, by consuming off abundant body fat. This is ordinary and people have advanced to fasting for shorter timespans—hours or days—without hindering wellbeing consequences. Body fat is only food vitality that has been put-away. If that you don't eat, your body will just "eat" its own fat for vitality.

Life is about parity. The great and the terrible, the yin

and the yang. The equivalent applies to eating and fasting. Fasting, all things considered, is essentially the other side of eating. If you are not eating, you are fasting. Here's the means by which it works. When we eat, more food vitality is ingested than can promptly be utilized. A portion of this vitality must be put-away for some time in the future. Insulin is the key hormone associated with the capacity of food vitality.

Insulin rises when we eat, assisting with putting away the overabundant vitality in two separate manners. Starches are separated into singular glucose (sugar) units, which can be connected into long ties to form glycogen, which is then put-away in the liver or muscle. There is, be that as it may, extremely constrained extra room for sugars; and once that is arrived at, the liver begins to transform the overabundance glucose into fat. This procedure is called lipogenesis (which means "making new fat").

A portion of this recently made fat is put-away in the liver, however its greater part is traded to other fat stores in the body. While this is an increasingly entangled procedure, there is practically no restriction to the measure of fat that can be made. In this way, two corresponding food vitality stockpiling frameworks exist in our bodies. One is effectively open yet with constrained extra room (glycogen), and the other is progressively hard to get to, however, it has practically boundless extra room (muscle versus fat).

The procedure goes backward when we don't eat (intermittent fasting). Insulin levels fall, flagging the body to begin consuming put-away vitality as no more is coming through food. Blood glucose falls, so the body should now haul glucose out of capacity to consume for vitality.   Glycogen is the most effectively available vitality source. It is separated into glucose particles to give vitality to the body's different cells. This can give enough vitality to control a significant part of the body's requirements for 24-36 hours. From that point onward, the body will fundamentally be separating fat for energy.

So, the body only truly exists in two states—the fed (insulin high) state and the fasted (insulin low) state. It is possible that we are either putting away food vitality (expanding stores), or we are consuming put-away vitality (diminishing stores). If that eating and fasting are adjusted, at that point there ought to be no net weight change. If we begin eating the moment we wake up, and don't stop until we rest, we invest practically the entirety of our energy in the fed state. After some time, we may put on weight, since we have not permitted our body at any point to consume put-away food energy.

To reestablish harmony or to get more fit, we may just need to build the measure of time spent consuming food energy. That's intermittent fasting. Basically, intermittent fasting permits the body to utilize its put-away vitality. All things considered that is what it is there for. The significant factor to comprehend is that there is nothing amiss. That is the way our bodies are structured. This is what hounds, felines, lions and bears do. It is humans' specialty.

If that you are eating each fourth hour, as is regularly prescribed, at that point your body will continually utilize the incoming food vitality. It should not consume a lot of muscle to fat ratio, assuming any. You may simply be putting away fat. Your body might be sparing it for when there is nothing to eat.

If that this occurs, you need balance. You need intermittent fasting.

What is intermittent fasting?

Intermittent fasting – isn't that starvation?

No. Fasting contrasts from starvation in one pivotal manner: control. Starvation is the automatic nonappearance of food for quite a while. This can prompt extreme misery or even death. It is neither conscious nor controlled.

Fasting is the deliberate retention of food for profound wellbeing, or different reasons. It's done by somebody who isn't underweight and in this way has enough put-away muscle to fat ratio to live off. Intermittent fasting done right shouldn't cause enduring, and surely never death.

With intermittent fasting, nourishment is effectively accessible, yet you decide not to eat it. This can be for any timeframe, from a couple of hours up to a couple of days or—with clinical supervision—even possibly more than seven days. You may start a fast whenever based on your personal preference, and you may end it freely as well. You can begin or stop a fast under any circumstances, with no explanation whatsoever.

Fasting has no standard term, as it is just the nonattendance of eating. Anytime that you are not eating, you are intermittently fasting. For instance, you may fast between meal and breakfast the following day, a time of around 12-14 hours. In that sense, intermittent fasting ought to be viewed as a part of regular life. Consider the expression "break fast". This refers to the meal that breaks your fast—which is done every day. As opposed to being a type of merciless and strange discipline, the English language certainly recognizes that fasting ought to be performed every day, regardless of whether it is just for a brief span.

Intermittent fasting isn't something irregular and inquisitive, rather, a part of ordinary, typical life. It is maybe the most established and most impressive dietary intercession imaginable. Yet, by one way or another, we have missed its capacity and disregarded its remedial potential.

Intermittent fasting is abandoning food for a specific timeframe. Fasting cycles change—some include fasting for somewhere in the range of 16-24 hours, and eating is confined to a specific window—from 12pm to 8pm, 11am to 7pm, and so on. Different methodologies prescribe eating typically for 5 days and seriously limiting calories on the other two days. This is known as the 5:2 eating routine.

Intermittent fasting (IF) is not quite the same as caloric

limitation (CR), which likewise gives a comparative record of medical advantages and shows guarantee in test animals at expanding our life expectancy. With caloric limitation, you're essentially eating less calories in a day. Intermittent fasting is frequently called an 'eating design' since it is increasingly about planning and when you eat. The particular planning of intermittent fasting affects certain hormonal procedures that advantage our wellbeing.

It Improves Wellbeing

Studies on intermittent fasting demonstrate that it can bring about weight reduction, fat decrease and an improved digestion, alongside improving insulin obstruction, which can assume a fundamental job in stoutness just as wellbeing. It sends our bodies into ketosis, which can upgrade weight reduction and furthermore offers a large group of extra advantages. When you're abandoning food for a specific timeframe, you may normally decrease calorie intake. In any case, individuals frequently think that it's simpler to follow IF as it consumes less calories and it doesn't include continually eating less at each meal, so they are bound to stay with it. Fasting periods likewise lessen late-night eating which such a significant number of us fall prey to.

CIRCADIAN RHYTHM

Advocates of intermittent fasting note that making an ordinary daily schedule and explicit planning around food encourages us to direct our circadian mood. It can assist us with taking advantage of our natural organic beat, prompting the correct arrival of hormones in the perfect sum, for example, insulin and development hormones. This can prompt a diminished danger of diabetes, improve our digestion, and assist us with keeping up a sound weight.

CARDIOVASCULAR HEALTH

Intermittent fasting can help decrease some cardiovascular hazard factors, for example, triglycerides, pulse and cholesterol, just as levels of C-receptive protein, a marker of aggravation.

Assimilation

Fasting can decidedly affect the microbiome (our settlement of gut microscopic animals that is basic to acceptable absorption, state of mind and insusceptibility), just as reinforce our intestinal hindrance and help bolster the gut's normal circadian mood. As a culture, we have a propensity for continually eating and nibbling—and this squeezes our stomach related tract. A time of fasting enables our bodies to finish their stomach-related procedures and gives us a rest, particularly at night when digestion might be slower.

INSULIN RESISTANCE + DIABETES

Studies show that IF can help improve insulin opposition, upgrade beta cells and can be a powerful eating design for individuals who have diabetes. What's more, IF can help with weight reduction—one of the significant hazard factors for diabetes.

Prevent Disease

Intermittent fasting has been known as an enemy of malignant growth impacts, as it can restrain the flagging pathways that prompt disease. It can likewise bring down the foundational aggravation related with disease hazard, restrain tumor development, and even improve the impacts of malignancy medications.

Get Rid of Irritation

Studies show that IF can decrease C-responsive protein levels, one of the significant pointers of irritation. It can likewise bring down ace fiery cytokines and invulnerable cells, as well as prevent oxidative pressure that can in the long run lead to irritation.

ATHLETIC PERFORMANCE

Intermittent fasting upgrades human development hormones that can assist us with consuming fat and forming muscle. Some evidence shows that IF can assist competitors with improving body arrangement and their general wellbeing.

Cerebrum HEALTH + ANTI-AGING

Analysts have investigated the impacts of IF on mind wellbeing and found that it can help limit oxidative pressure that prompts cerebrum maturing and secures the sensory system, as well as help prevent neurological diseases like Alzheimer's and Parkinson's.

Disadvantages of Intermittent Fasting

A few things to know about if you're keen on attempting intermittent fasting.

It's hard: While a few people find IF simpler than steady caloric limitation, that doesn't mean it's simple. You truly should be a cognizant eater and fight the temptation to eat, despite the fact that you may feel hungry. There aren't a ton of dietary principles: Intermittent fasters are urged to eat a solid eating routine, however there aren't explicit standards about what's ideal. That implies that any food could be included, and a few fixings or food sources aren't the best decisions.

Voraciously consuming food: Prolonged limitation may prompt gorging or eating lousy foods.

Enthusiastic components: IF can be extreme, sincerely and socially. It can likewise be a trigger for individuals with confused eating designs.

Hormonal elements: If you experience the ill effects of any sort of hormonal unevenness, fasting could be a fuel to that imbalanced fire and cause a decline of side effects. Some state that it's really declining before it improves, however that by itself could be an impediment.

WHAT ARE THE BENEFITS OF INTERMITTENT FASTING?

Research on intermittent fasting is still in its early stages. A great deal of studies have just been carried out on animals. Be that as it may, the potential advantages are promising.

INTERMITTENT FASTING BENEFITS

WEIGHT LOSS

How about we be genuine here, this is the main reason individuals are taking a gander at intermittent fasting. Individuals need to get thinner and individuals need easy routes to do it. You can get thinner with intermittent fasting BUT it will be joined with a solid eating regimen (and exercise will help). Truly, you won't get more fit if you eat precisely the same foods you're now eating just in a shorter timeframe.

INTERMITTENT FASTING BENEFITS

ANTI-AGING

We're all getting older. Every. Single. Day. It sucks, I know. Yet, in light of the fact that we're getting more seasoned doesn't mean we like to look or act older.

Anti-aging applies to something other than your appearance. Certainly, I'd like to resemble a 20-year-old once more. Be that as it may, I'd likewise prefer to feel like a 20-year-old once more. Those little pains that begin showing up in your mid-late thirties, don't you wish you could dispose of them?

BOOSTS BRAIN HEALTH

A solid mind is about something other than preventing dementia or similar brain diseases. Mind wellbeing influences your memory and body. Your mind controls you both physically and intellectually.

HEART HEALTH

A sound heart is a solid you. There are numerous sorts of heart issues, including circulatory strain, pulse, cholesterol and the sky is the limit from there. Intermittent fasting can assist with improving all markers of heart wellbeing.

CANCER

Malignancy is a shockingly common horrendous disease. More examinations are required (particularly in people) yet early investigations of animals show that intermittent fasting could help prevent malignancy. Extremely restricted, yet encouraging, examiners propose that fasting can help lessen the need for chemotherapy in malignant growth patients.

REDUCED INSULIN RESISTANCE

What is insulin obstruction? It's the point at which your body doesn't deal with insulin appropriately. This is the main source of Type 2 Diabetes.

Would you like to have Type 2 Diabetes? Definitely not.

Intermittent Fasting could altogether diminish glucose and insulin, in men. There's one investigation of ladies that shows compounded glucose. It was a small and short examination, at the same time, ladies ought to know that they may not share this advantage.

WHAT ARE THE DISADVANTAGES OF INTERMITTENT FASTING?

There are two impediments to intermittent fasting.

The first is brief: Beginning. It's difficult to begin. You'll get ravenous—from the outset. However, in the long run, you'll adapt and it turns out to be simple. You eat less frequently and less food which implies less time considering what to eat and where and how. It implies you're investing less energy getting ready food. If you can get over the underlying obstacle of being ravenous, it leaves. You quit feeling hungry constantly.

The subsequent one is reliant on what you're eating. Intermittent fasting can cause shaky glucose levels. If you've been fasting for a few hours and eat an enormous meal, substantial in carbs, your glucose will spike far up. It will gradually go down as you fast. Eating a low carb diet can essentially decrease (or dispense with) this burden. If you're not eating a low carb diet, at that point, ensure you're eating adjusted meals. Try not to pig out on carbs at the same time and you'll relieve a great deal of the hazard.

WHO SHOULDN'T TRY INTERMITTENT FASTING?

Everybody should check with a medicinal services specialist before starting intermittent fasting. Notwithstanding, it's particularly discouraged for the following individuals:

- Pregnant Women

- Anybody with a background marked by dietary issues

- Individuals with diabetes

- A person with another good dieting plan and

exercise

Who Should Be Careful Or Avoid It?

Intermittent fasting is absolutely not for everybody. If you're underweight or have a background marked by dietary issues, you ought not fast without counseling with a wellbeing specialist first. In these cases, it very well may be absolutely unsafe.

Frequency of Intermittent Fasting

Now that you know how to do intermittent fasting, then another question comes to mind: How many times weekly should you fast?

The answer varies with different individuals. Some people fast weekly while others prefer the monthly fasting period. If you're new to fasting, start with a modest schedule, keep practicing the fast, you can put your schedule on a weekly or monthly basis. If your body adjusts well, aim for a frequent weekly schedule.

There's no wrong answer here. Pay keen interest to how your body reacts to your fasting schedule and regulate it as needed. Keep in mind that a lot of changes can take place in your body while you fast. In addition, you may need to twist your timetable to allow for social gatherings, holidays, and physical activity or contests.

CHAPTER FOUR

DIFFERENT TYPES OF FASTING

PROTOCOL

Please note, before you start any type of fasting, it is advisable you consult your doctor to know the type that is best for you. Ulcer patients and the likes should not be involved in total abstinence from food. In a nutshell, don't go through fasting without doing proper medical checkups.

DIFFERENT TYPES OF FASTING PROTOCOL

Below are what you need to do before you commence fasting, this is important especially when the fasting will last for several days.

1) Different strokes for different folks they say. There are people who believe you are to go without water while you fast while there are those who believe water is essential while fasting. But you must check the kind of life you live while you fast. Ensure you maintain a good lifestyle, for instance, walking under the early morning sun for some minutes, taking enough water and getting at least eight hours of sleep while you fast. However, don't fast to stay indoors all day and

shutdown your personal hygiene, fast to keep yourself fit and live a healthy life.

2) Getting to know how healthy you are medically is the second major prerequisite before commencing a fast. Ask yourself these questions:

- What is my blood sugar level?
- Am I an ulcer patient?
- What are my allergies?
- How do I feel whenever I undergo fasting?

Intermittent fasting is a model of fasting and eating over some period of time. It is not defined by some meals, though it can also mean observing nutritional ketosis during times of eating.

Intermittent fasting can be used occasionally or whenever the need arises. You may even like to mix and match throughout the year, practicing some daily. It can also be an annual routine or done on a monthly basis. Different methods that entail research, trial and error have proven that intermittent fasting is effective, the good news is, you can find the one that suits you best here.

We have put different types of intermittent fasting

together to help you choose the one that best suits you.

Fasting is currently one of the ways to lose weight and listed below are the three major types.

THREE TYPES OF FASTING:

The three main form of fasting are: calorie control, nutrient restriction, and seasonal eating.

CALORIE CONTROL FASTS

The primary type of fast is a calorie control fast. This is what most people think about when they hear the term "fasting". It is simply going without food for a particular time. Calorie controlled fasts are usually done between 18-48 hours. To use this type of fast effectively, ensure you have taken in the number of required calories the days before the commencement of the fast. Then pick a day after you are sure your calories are at the right numbers, start by eating meal early, and fast for the designated time. In the fasting period, only consume water and keep activity levels low to support the internal part of the body.

MACRO NUTRIENT RESTRICTION FASTS

This type of fast entails controlling a certain

macronutrient (the three macronutrients are proteins, carbohydrates, and fats). Typically, these fasts boost protein. Athletes undergo this type of fast a lot and it usually gives higher protein while it cleanses the guts. Moreover, in this period, athletes consume only high-quality fat containing meals, carbohydrates, and they must eat cooked vegetables for 2-3 days in thirty days. The decline in protein consumption will give the gut a break and healing. Have in mind that it is still vital to have minimal activity during this type of fast.

SEASONAL EATING

Decades ago during winter, we loved to eat fattier meats and tubers, while fruits and shredded meats used to be eaten during summer. It is wise to eat only foods available during that time of the year. While our continental food access is great, some nations around northern latitudes wouldn't get to see ripe papaws/bananas/apples in January. Seasonal or occasional eating follows the theory of personalized nutrition based on your environment; knowing what would be available at an exact time of the year are key factors to note if you want to experience seasonal fasting.

Alternate day fasting

As the name implies, this involves fasting every other day. On fasting days, you can only consume meals of 500 calories, or complete fasting (without calories). On other days, you can eat normally (as with all fasting, nutritional ketosis is advisable at this time). Long-term, this is an intense method of fasting, and might not be sustainable over time.

Spontaneous fasting/Skipping meals

This is highly recommended for anyone who is on the fence about intermittent fasting, or feels overwhelmed by setting controlled fasting times.

This is a mild introduction to intermittent fasting, which is achieved by your lifestyle and body. It is the best for those who don't like to undergo regimented diets, or get discouraged if they don't meet the criteria of their diet.

Intermittent Fasting Methods

There are a few unique methods for undergoing intermittent fasting—all of which include dividing the day or week into eating and fasting periods.

During the fasting time frames, you eat either next to nothing or nothing at all.

These are the most well-known strategies:

The 16/8 strategy: Also called the Leangains convention, it includes skipping breakfast and confining your day by day eating period to 8 hours, for example, 1–9 p.m. At that point you fast for 16 hours in the middle.

Eat-Stop-Eat: This includes fasting for 24 hours, on more than one occasion per week, for instance by not having meal on one day until meal the following day.

The 5:2 eating routine: With this strategy, you devour just 500–600 calories on two non-successive days of the week, yet eat typically the other 5 days.

By diminishing your calorie consumption, these strategies should cause weight reduction as long as you don't remunerate by eating significantly more during the eating time frames. Numerous individuals find the 16/8 strategy to be the least complex, generally maintainable and most straightforward to adhere to. It's likewise the most famous.

There are a few unique approaches to intermittent fasting. Every one of them splits the day or week into eating and fasting periods.

SIX WAYS OF FASTING

Whether you're just starting your IF program or you've tried fasting before but couldn't sustain it for long-term, it turns out there are several ways of fasting, modified to fit your lifestyle and behavior.

1: Omit a Meal

If you've never tried intermittent fasting, here is the best guide to start. By explanation, intermittent fasting simply means going for a lengthened period of time without meal.

The best time frame is around16/8 for intermittent fasting.

Most people could get related benefits just from skipping breakfast, lunch or meal. Try omitting a meal plan and see if you can work toward the 16-hours fasting, 8-hour eating gap. You might just start to feel amazing.

2: Fast Within a Daily Window

Like the 16/8 technique, there are other eating programs (known as feeding windows) you can try out.

The fact is—you're already doing this to some point because you fast every day between meal and breakfast daily, hopefully you don't eat at midnight.

Here's what it is:

If you eat breakfast around 8 a.m. and your last meal of the day was at 5 p.m., it means you ate within a 9-hour period. However, you will need to fast for the 15 hours left in the day.

The next reasonable step to planned intermittent fasting is widening your fasting window and lessening your feeding window.

You might want to attempt the 16/8 method, which might look exactly like eating all of your foods between 10 a.m. and 6 p.m.

Another illustration is the 18/6 scheme. With this method, you will be increasing your fasting window to 18 hours, which might mean consumption of meals between noon and 6 p.m.

This is the best place to start if you're passionate about IF, but not set to go through a whole day without having something to eat. It's very easy to adapt to your unique timetable and lifestyle.

3: Alternate-Day Fasting

Alternate-day fasting is exactly what it is, you will need to fast for a whole day, then eat normally the next day.

Here is how it should be:

- Monday: Fasting

- Tuesday: Eat as usual

- Wednesday: Fasting

- Thursday: Eat as usual

- And so on.

According to the knowledge available on alternate day fasting, you can take one of these two methods:

1. You can fast solely on fasting days, while you only sip water, or

2. You can eat little meals up to 25% of your usual caloric intake. This equals about 500-600 calories for most people. Here's the good news—sugar or starches should not be added to the 25%.

4: Fat Fasting

Fat fasting is a great choice for those who are already in ketosis or want to get into ketosis swiftly. It's also a thing of joy if you've been doing keto for a while and eventually lose weight.

Moreover, you should not do fat fasting beyond 2-4 days—it should not exceed five days.

Here's how it goes:

- You should eat 80-90% of your calories from fat only for 2-4 days.

- You can limit caloric ingestion to 1000-1200 calories daily.

- Breaking this up into 200-250-calorie meals all day is also advisable.

- Fat fasting seems not to have an eating and fasting window involved, as long as you're engaging in intense fat diet consumption. If you can imagine yourself eating avocados and spoonfuls of cocoa butter for three days, you might just be fasting this way.

5: The combatant Diet

One of the major benefits of caloric restriction is the combatant diet. First organized by a man named Ori Hofmekler, a former representative of the Israeli Special Force, the diet was meant to emulate the diets of ancient combatants.

Apparently, these combatants kept their minds sharp and their waistlines trim by eating very little throughout the day and eating one big meal as meal. Those that take ketogenic related meals should take low-carb veggies and keto snacks during the day.

You can also refrain from food entirely throughout the day and eat one big meal at night.

But since small meals are "allowed here" before night fall, this method can be easier than forgoing food for the whole day. Just be sure not to consume any food late at night, which can cause stomach upset and digestive disorders.

6: Eat-stop-Eat, or a 24-Hour total Fast

This form of fasting is—as the name implies—a total 24-hour fast.

That means, for 24-hours, you only drink water if you

want to stay in a complete fasting state. Though it is still healthy to consume non-caloric beverages like non-sugary juice (homemade), coffee (rich in cocoa) and tea. You're permitted to do it the way you desire.

The timetable of this intermittent fasting plan depends on how you want it.

You could commerce after meal. For instance, Wednesday evening, fast the following day, and have meal on that Thursday evening.

As long as you don't take in any calories for an entire 24 hours, you're all right.

This can be the best way to get into ketosis more speedily, but a 24-hour fast is also very demanding for most people. If you're a learner, you might want to start with a more restrained 12- to 16-hour fast to build up a tolerance.

How It Affects Your Cells and Hormones

When you fast, a few things occur in your body on the cell and atomic level. For instance, your body modifies hormone levels to make put-away muscle versus fat increasingly available.

Your cells likewise start significant repair procedures

and change the statement of qualities. Here are a few changes that happen in your body when you fast:

Human Growth Hormone (HGH): The degrees of development hormones soar, expanding as much as 5-overlap. This has benefits for fat loss and muscle gain, to give some examples.

Insulin: Insulin affectability improves and levels of insulin drop significantly. Lower insulin levels make put-away muscle to fat ratio increasingly open.

Cell fix: When fasting, your cells start cell repair forms. This includes autophagy, where cells overview and expel old and broken proteins that develop inside cells.

Quality articulation: There are changes in the capacity of qualities identified with life span and security against ailment.

These adjustments in hormone levels, cell capacity and quality articulation are liable for the medical advantages of intermittent fasting.

When you fast, human development hormone levels go up and insulin levels go down. Your body's cells likewise change the outflow of qualities and start significant cell repair forms.

CHAPTER FIVE

MYTHS ABOUT INTERMITTENT FASTING

Weight reduction is the most widely recognized reason behind individuals attempting intermittent fasting.

By causing you to eat less meals, intermittent fasting can prompt a programmed decrease in calorie consumption. Moreover, intermittent fasting changes hormone levels to encourage weight reduction.

Notwithstanding bringing down insulin and expanding development hormone levels, it builds the arrival of the fat consuming hormone, norepinephrine (noradrenaline). In view of these adjustments in hormones, momentary fasting may expand your metabolic rate by 3.6–14%.

By helping you eat less and consume less calories, intermittent fasting causes weight reduction by changing the two sides of the calorie condition. Studies show that intermittent fasting can be an extremely incredible weight reduction apparatus.

A 2014 survey study found that this eating method can cause 3–8% weight reduction within 3–24 weeks, which is a huge sum, contrasted with most weight reduction methods.

As per a similar report, individuals additionally lost 4–7% of their midriff circuit, showing a noteworthy loss of unwanted stomach fat that develops around your organs and causes disease.

Another examination demonstrated that intermittent fasting causes less muscle loss than the more standard strategy for consistent calorie limitation.

In any case, remember that the fundamental explanation behind its prosperity is that intermittent fasting causes you to eat less calories, generally speaking. If you gorge and eat large amounts of food during your eating periods, you may not lose any weight whatsoever.

Individuals who need to be cautious about fasting and exercise as a rule include those with insulin opposition, diabetes, metabolic disorder, or other wellbeing conditions that influence blood glucose levels, as exercise in the fasted state could cause glucose to drop. In any case, all in all, ordinary exercise is connected to glucose control, it simply must be done carefully.

Exercise is additionally conceivable during alternate day fasts, which include more prominent caloric limitation (CR) every other day for a set number of days (usually 2–3 days in a given week). One randomized, controlled investigation of 83 solid members, who ate a meal comparable to 25% of vitality needs on their fasting days, somewhere in the range of 12:00pm and 2:00pm, and practiced on stationary bicycles or curved machines for 25 minutes at 60% of their objective pulse, in weeks 1–4 as long as 40 minutes at 75% of their objective pulse, didn't encounter any unfavorable impacts. Truth be told, the members who occupied with physical action in addition to CR encountered an abatement in weight and abdomen periphery with no loss of fit bulk. Moreover, the "terrible cholesterol" (LDL-C) went down and the "great cholesterol" (HDL-C) went up.

What you eat when you're fasting matters significantly more if you're including exercise. A few sorts of activity ought to be trailed by more protein. Protein has appeared to increment myofibrillar protein amalgamation, which adds to muscle development.

Research additionally proposes that the body depends more on fat for fuel than starches after this sort of activity in a fasted state.

As usual, you ought to counsel with your human services specialist, particularly if you take meds or live with a constant wellbeing condition, to check whether joining exercise during your fast is suitable for you.

What the entirety of this exploration means might be essentially abridged as:

- Exercise can work inside most fasting conventions.

If that ideal execution is your objective during a fasting period, spare high-power exercises for after you've eaten. After an exercise, especially including high-power preparing or opposition preparing, when you do eat once more, eat protein. You may think you need food to fuel your exercises, however you are incorrect.

As of late, the counsel that proposes stacking up on starches before exercise has had doubts raised about it. Truly, devouring carbs before exercise can build execution in specific fields like running and sports that utilize power developments, however it likewise prevents the body from utilizing put-away muscle versus fat for vitality, which implies you are less inclined to receive the revealed fat consuming rewards.

In this way, if you exercise to remain slim, going 'fasted' is the more viable choice.

What does fasting mean?

Through the span of the day you go through fed and fasted states. The fed state goes on for around four to six hours after your last meal, during which your body discharges insulin to bring down your glucose. Proteins and fats are consumed by the digestive system, and glucose is moved to the muscles to be utilized as vitality (glycogen).

Six hours in the wake of eating you enter the fasted state. Glucagon is discharged to keep your glucose at ordinary levels. Your body begins to separate (fat) tissue into free unsaturated fats, which would then be able to be changed over into a type of vitality known as ketone bodies. In layman's terms, you're consuming fat for vitality.

When you begin eating, the procedure is ended.

Insulin presently restrains the breakdown of unsaturated fats, driving your body to consume the sugars you've recently ingested. The fat consuming stage is finished.

Things being what they are, this all bodes well. When food wasn't as promptly accessible as it is today, clutching put-away muscle to fat ratio was urgent for our endurance. We developed to keep going quite a while between meals.

Today, food is in practically steady stockpile—yet our bodies are still physiologically equivalent to how they were a huge number of years before. If we eat throughout the day, we never tap into our bodies' normal capacity to consume put-away muscle to fat ratio for vitality.

Studies show that exercise in the fasted as contrasted to the non-fasted state builds the dependence on fat and accordingly lessens the dependence on starch as fuel during exercise, with a few distributions indicating that fasted practice oxidizes (consumes) around 20-30pc progressive fat.

If you're practicing to get more fit, it's an easy decision.

Instructions to actualize it

The hypothesis behind fasted practice is solid—however for any individual who's gone through decades turning out on an overwhelming carb load, it means a major difference in propensity. Which is the reason I recommend beginning your fasting with very delicate, vigorous exercises, for example, strolling, running, swimming or cycling. At first, your exercises will feel much harder than before, yet rapidly your body will turn out to be progressively effective as your muscles figure out how to utilize less glycogen and consume fat for fuel.

When you become accustomed to it, you may discover there's no going back.

It's additionally critical to take note of this if you will do an especially strenuous exercise, you ought to eat some carbs beforehand. That way, you'll prevent your glucose levels from dropping excessively low, which can cause dazedness and sickness.

So would it be a good idea for me to stay away from carbs totally?

While I prescribe practicing fasting, that doesn't mean you ought to consistently remain off carbs. For sure, issues can emerge with intermittent fasting when joined with low carbs from eating less. The issue here is that you can diminish the body's capacity to use starch. At last, the objective ought to be 'metabolic adaptability'—that is, to take action to utilize both carbs and fat as and when required. Two vitality stores are superior to one.

Be vital with your starch consumption. Eat more on your preparation days and less on your rest days.

Would I be able to have anything before a workout?

Yes—to a degree. Taking something light like green tea helps with digestion.

I ought to likewise say that you should consistently drink water—previously, during, and after a workout.

The Pros of Combining Intermittent Fasting and Keto

Pros: Your craving diminishes

Supplanting carbs with fat on a keto diet makes hunger decline, perhaps because of movements in craving controlling hormones. When you're fat-adjusted on the keto diet and your craving is lower than ordinary, you'll most likely discover the fasting bit of IF simpler.

Pros: You may get in shape faster

The controlled calories from the short eating window, in addition to the way that you're utilizing fat for vitality, may imply that you may lose more weight in a shorter timeframe. While this can be an advantage for those hoping to get in shape, research proposes that weight reduction from IF and keto may not be any better in the long haul contrasted with a low-calorie diet.

Pros: You arrive at ketosis faster

The ketogenic diet confines carbs so the body changes to fat for fuel. Simultaneously, fasting causes the body's glycogen levels to exhaust, so the mix of the two weight control plans together resembles a most optimized plan of attack to ketosis. This can help moderate the "keto influence," an especially frightful manifestation of the change into ketosis.

The Cons of Combining Intermittent Fasting and Ketosis

Con: Keto doesn't ensure great wellbeing

Fouled up, keto can at present be unfortunate, and IF doesn't change that. Not at all like what numerous individuals see it to be, the ketogenic diet isn't intended to be loaded with cheddar, eggs, and bacon. To help dodge increments in LDL cholesterol, the keto diet ought to be founded on, for the most part, unsaturated fats from sources, for example, avocados, nuts, and olive oils.

Con: It might influence athletic execution

While IF may help lessen fat stores while protecting bulk, the amazingly low carb level of the ketogenic diet has been shown to contrarily influence athletic execution. This may not be the situation with everybody, except sugars, not fat, are as yet viewed as the best wellspring of fuel for competitors.

Con: It's difficult

It's a great deal of limitation. A great many people would consider the ketogenic diet genuinely prohibitive all alone, with its amazingly low carb limits.

Indeed, due to the degree of limitation, many people can't adhere to extremely low carb limits as long as possible. Including a layer of time limitations on the keto diet might be an excessive amount to deal with. What's more, the advantages of these weight control plans are available just during the time that you're on them; they will in general vanish once you return to your typical dietary patterns.

Combining Keto and IF

We have referenced more than once that fasting is overly well known among individuals who are additionally following a ketogenic diet. There might be some strong hypothesis behind this.

Truth be told, eating a ketogenic high-fat low-carb diet will make fasting simpler and increasingly sensible. This is on the grounds that a keto diet will assist you with losing weight, which will improve your capacity to play out an all-encompassing fast without feeling dormant, discouraged, or intolerably eager.

Keto diet and intermittent fasting both have the equivalent metabolic objectives—train the body to productively consume fat for vitality and get into a condition of ketosis. The two regimens do this by exhausting glucose and bringing down insulin levels in the body. Another bit of leeway of joining keto with intermittent fasting is that IF may assist you with getting into ketosis significantly faster and maybe accomplish higher ketone levels.

Keto and IF Diet Plan

Perhaps you're contemplating attempting the keto diet or exploring different avenues regarding fasting. Maybe you're as of now doing both.

The keto diet and intermittent fasting are two well known, powerful approaches to get in shape rapidly. The two strategies bring upon comparable changes in the body: more ketones, lower glucose and, in any event, improved state of mind and mental lucidity. Both additionally call for less snacks, however the keto diet confines which snacks you eat while intermittent fasting limits when you nibble.

It's common to explore different avenues regarding either the keto diet or intermittent fasting (however it's in every case better to consult a specialist first). In any case, how safe is it to combine the two? To start with, we should investigate what both of these weight reduction approaches do to the body, and how those procedures may associate.

The keto diet

In basic terms, ketosis is a metabolic procedure wherein the body begins consuming fat for fuel rather than sugar (glucose). Ketosis happens normally when the body needs more glucose to use as vitality, so it rather goes to put-away fats, which it changes over into ketones that are dispersed through blood to muscles and other tissue. The keto diet triggers this procedure by requiring an eating routine high in fat and low in starches, which brings about lower levels of glucose and insulin.

These days, it's difficult to start a diet culture without knowing about the keto diet or some types of intermittent fasting.

It is becoming a popular eating style among celebrities around the world, most of them want to look fit and slim down so that they glow when they appear on the screen. If you are a fan of Instagram, you will see celebrities praising this fasting method. However, we have those that do both keto diet and intermittent fasting religiously—but the question is, is it very effective? And more significantly, is it healthy to do the keto diet and intermittent fasting together? The information you will see below will lecture you about how to effectively combine intermittent fasting and keto diet with little or no side effects. If you also want to know whether or not you should try them together, the information below will give you the answers.

What exactly is the keto diet, anyway?

The ketogenic diet is a macronutrient-controlled pattern of eating where the greater part of the calories you eat come from fat, while the remaining comes from a modest amount of protein with little to no carbohydrate. In the main time, it means saying goodbye to fruit and pasta, and welcoming items like steak and eggs with both hands.

This high-fat, low-carb diet encourages the body to use fat for energy instead of sugars. When your body does not have enough carbs to sustain everyday activity, the liver breaks down fat into ketones, which can then be used as energy. This metabolic process is called ketosis—that's where the phrase "going keto" comes from.

Research reveals that the keto diet can have many health benefits. It's been proven to boost weight loss, develop brain functions, and reduce blood sugar levels. It has aided many people who have suffered from obesity and diabetes. However, eating in this way can be really challenging.

Kristen Mancinelli, who wrote 'Ketogenic Diet', believes "People don't usually style their plate around fat. What it means is, everyone should indeed eat 25 grams of carbohydrates a day, especially those that contain non-starchy vegetables like broccoli or lettuce. Though it is easier said than done because it's not what we're used to, everyone should try it."

WHICH IS THE BEST FOR WOMEN?

There is some proof that intermittent fasting may not be as advantageous for ladies for what it's worth for men. For instance, one examination indicated that it improved insulin affectability in men, however compounded glucose control in ladies.

In spite of the fact that human investigations on this point are inaccessible, concentrates in rodents have discovered that intermittent fasting can make female rodents withered, masculinized, barren and cause them to miss cycles.

There are various episodic reports of ladies whose menstrual period halted when they began doing IF and returned to ordinary when they continued their past eating design. Thus, ladies ought to be cautious with intermittent fasting. They ought to follow separate rules, such as slipping into the practice.

SHOULD WOMEN FAST?

Possibly. In any case, perhaps not. Ladies may have motivation to be more cautious than men. Studies on the impacts of intermittent fasting on ladies are incredibly restricted. There may be issues with intermittent fasting causing more regrettable glucose, barrenness, and amenorrhea (no period) in certain ladies.

HOW TO CHOOSE YOUR FASTING HOURS/METHOD?

Few out of every odd technique for fasting will work for you. There are a few famous techniques for intermittent fasting: The 16/8 Method (otherwise known as Leangains): Fast for 16 hours and eat for 8 hours, consistently.

Eat-stop-eat Method: 24-hour fasts on more than one occasion per week.

The 5:2 eating regimen (otherwise known as the Fast Diet): Eat ordinarily for 5 days, "fast" (eat around 500 calories) 2 days.

Crescendo Method

12-16 hours of fasting, 2-3 days every week. For more descriptive information about the most famous techniques, look at Intermittent Fasting Methods.

If you find yourself in a discussion about dieting or weight loss, odds are you'll hear of the ketogenic, keto, or similar means of dieting.

That's because the keto diet has turned to one of the most trendy methods globally to shed surplus weight and improve health.

Studies have shown that adopting this low-carb, fat concentrated diet supports fat loss and may develop certain conditions like type 2 diabetes while there is cognitive decline.

CHAPTER SIX

INTERMITTENT FASTING AND

KETOGENIC DIET

Here come the benefits of using intermittent fasting and keto collectively.

If you include IF into your keto arrangement, one big plus you may notice is that you will attain ketosis faster. Why? Fasting helps your body to move its fuel storage away from carbs and onto fats, which is, of course, the same method keto uses to enable you to shed weight. Plus, your body burns fat for power when you fast— another keto-friendly conception. It usually takes a couple of days for your body to initiate weight loss mode on keto, so feasibly, intermittent fasting can help you to shed weight from all parts of the body.

Is it healthy to simultaneously do keto and intermittent fasting?

It is a question that can be answered independently. It really depends solely on you. For example, if you take certain drugs, fasting may not be harmless. If you have blood sugar troubles or are on blood sugar lowering drugs, any of these diets could be really dangerous or even fatal.

Clearly, if you're pregnant, any form of weight loss diet will not be right for you. Likewise, if you have a chronic health status, you need to refrain for some period or you may need to consult your doctor for this.

It's really important to talk to your doctor in details about keto and IF. A research study from the University of British Columbia discovered that the effortless act of taking advantage of a cheat day while on keto means you consume small meals that contain not more than 75 grams of glucose daily which can potentially harm your blood vessels. It is just a way of saying the combination of keto and IF is not good for everyone's health. The mix of sugar and high-fat, low-carb could also lead to a fatal status. Furthermore, calorie constraint could lead to complications in terms of the general well-being of your long-term health. The right route is, profile your health status and tell your medical consultant/nutritionist to analyze for you before commencing IF and keto together.

How do you combine intermittent fasting and keto?

Here are some guidelines on how to get the best out

of your IF-keto regimen.

Identify your overall intention.

Concentrate on meeting your caloric requirements to stay healthy. Ensure you're getting the right quantity of protein spaced throughout the phase of time that you are eating on IF, because there are restrictions to how much protein the body can take up and use at a given time. You also have to be certain that the required amount of vitamins and minerals are being met as well. You'll also need to reflect on how much fiber and fluids are required; it is doable if you're ready to lose weight.

Go slowly.

A 2018 research from the Johns Hopkins suggests that irregular fasting could be part of a healthy way of life, though physicians advise patients to steadily increase the time and frequency of the fasting era over the period of several months, instead of "doing cold turkey at all time."

Eat on time.

Painstakingly control the hours of the day when you

eat to around 10 a.m. to 6 pm, or 9 a.m. to 5 p.m. It's better to fast when you are near bedtime. But can you do this?

Book appointment with a dietitian.

Combining these plans (IF and keto) is often thriving when you work with an expert. "People underrate the result having a dietician in their circle can bring. Dieticians know the merits and demerits of keeping people safe, and having a dietician can be a game changer for you. A certified dietitian can help you circumvent eating disorder behavior, analyze your body image for you and assist you in balancing a dietary model that you can stick with long term—and most importantly, they help you meet your fitness goals."

Imagine sitting down to a balanced meal and consuming as much as you desire. Take a look at how you feel when is time to eat some piles of mild sautéed broccoli, some handful of poached white fish and a beet-arugula salad with a sprinkling of feta cheese. Imagine concluding your meal and not eating anything else … until noon the following day.

Seem like an organized fantasy? It isn't, though you

can't be blamed for thinking it might be. The world is obsessed with crunchy chips, soft breads, sky-high cakes and vanilla ice creams. If you're one of those to whom that list still calls, though you passionately wish it wouldn't, that's okay.

Imagine you could finally stop consuming unhealthy foods and overeating, dump those extra pounds and obesity, and eat the right food as its meant to be consumed? Healthy living gives energy, this will make you get back to living the life of your dreams, you don't need to overfeed or eat everything you see.

Well, the gist is, both intermittent fasting and the ketogenic make you live a healthy life. Changing not only the foods you consume but the way your body utilizes them is key. Many people already enjoy the opportunities of keto, and are now wondering how to take it to the next phase.

This segment will reveal methods of applying intermittent fasting, popularly called (IF), into your keto eating program.

While a lot of studies show both ways of eating independently, not much has been written on how to use them without them being harmful to you.

Let's take a quick look at what both the IF and keto are and how to use them together. Whether you currently follow keto and have interest in adding fasting to your toolkit, or haven't done any of these and keep wondering how they meet, then sit back and relax because this segment is meant for you.

Ketogenic Diet fundamentals

The keto diet is known to be very low in carbs, with intense fat and modest in protein.

When following a ketogenic diet, carbs are usually minimized to go below 50 grams per day.

Fats should swap with the majority of cut carbs and deliver around 75% of your total calorie consumption.

Proteins most times account for about 20% of energy needs, while carbs are usually limited to 5%.

This carb decline forces your body to depend on fats for its primary energy source instead of glucose—a process called ketosis.

While in ketosis, your body spends ketones—molecules formed in the liver from fats when glucose is inadequate—as another fuel source.

Though fat is always avoided for its high calorie content, studies reveal that ketogenic diets are notably more helpful at promoting weight loss than low-fat diets.

In addition, keto diets lessen hunger and boost satiety, which can be particularly useful when trying to shed weight.

WHY YOU SHOULD DO BOTH AND FOR HOW LONG?

The ketogenic diet is the type where the body is transformed from using glucose as its main energy molecule and starts to use ketones instead. Both can be used to power the body by engaging in some daily mission which can be thinking and movement, though most people prefer using diets to gain glucose to doing activities like endurance trekking.

Glucose is always accessible in the form of carbs, from grains, and fruit, to vegetables and processed sugar. When we eat any of these diets, the body readily processes them into glucose and dumps them into the bloodstream, which are then conveyed around the body with the aids of insulin for use in different tasks. Surplus glucose is taken up and kept as fat. The fats that are kept are not used up, because glucose is constantly being added to the system.

The ketogenic diet excludes carbohydrates, and therefore glucose, from the program. Your body still wants energy, so it will instead prefer to produce fat—keep energy. However, the liver will start processing the fat, producing ketones that can be used instead of glucose.

Moreover, whenever fat storage decreases in your body, ensure you take foods that contain glucose, but avoid taking them excessively. Thus far, keto has proven to be very helpful in dealing with obesity, reducing cholesterol and assisting people in maintaining a much higher level of good health.

Ketogenic Diet Meal Plan

Switching over to a ketogenic diet can appear overwhelming, but it doesn't have to be complicated.

Your aim should be on dipping carbs while escalating the fat and protein content of meals and snacks.

In order to attain ketosis and remain in a state of ketosis, carbs must be controlled.

While certain people might only attain ketosis by eating less than 20 grams of carbs daily, others may be successful with an amplified carb intake.

Generally, the lesser your carbohydrate intake, the easier it is to achieve and stay in ketosis.

This is because getting used to keto-friendly meals and avoiding stuff rich in carbs is the best way to effectively lose weight while using the ketogenic method.

Keto-Friendly Meals (RECIPES)

When observing a ketogenic diet, meals and snacks should revolve around the following staple:

- **Eggs:** Pastured, natural whole eggs make the best pick.

- **Poultry:** Chicken, meat, and turkey.

- **Fatty fish:** Salmon gotten from the wild, herring and mackerel.

- **Meat:** Beef that are herbivores, white/red meat, pork, organ meats and bison.

- **100% dairy:** Yogurt, margarine and cream.

- **Full-fat cheese:** Cheddar, creamy mozzarella, ointment cheese, brie, goat and cheese.

- **Nuts and seeds:** Macadamia nuts, groundnut, almonds, walnuts, pumpkin seeds, peanuts and flaxseeds.

- **Nut butter:** Organic peanut, almond and cashew margarine.

- **Healthy fats:** Coconut/sesame/avocado oil, and coconut butter.

- **Avocados:** A complete avocado can be added to roughly any food or snack.

- **Non-starchy vegetables:** Greens, lettuce, broccoli, tomatoes, mushrooms, carrots, and peppers.

- **Condiments:** Salt, spices, pepper, vinegar, herbs, lemon juice, fresh foods.

Items to Avoid

Do away with foods rich in carbs while observing a keto diet.

The following foods should be controlled:

- **Bread and baked items:** White scorched bread, complete wheat bread, crackers, spring roll, cookies, and doughnuts.

- **Sweets and sugary confectionaries:** Sugar, frost cream, chocolate, maple syrup, agave syrup and coconut sugar.

- **Sweetened beverages:** Soda, juice, sugared teas and sports or excessive energy drinks.

- **Pasta:** Spaghetti, macaroni, and noodles.

- **Grains and grain foodstuffs:** Wheat, tortillas, rice, oats, and some breakfast cereals.

- **Starchy vegetables:** Ordinary potatoes or sweet potatoes, butternut squash/mash, corn, peas and pumpkin.

- **Beans and legumes:** Especially black beans, chickpeas, lentils and kidney beans.

- **Fruit:** Citrus, water melon, grapes, bananas, and pineapple.

- **High-carb delicacy:** Barbecue meat/fish, sweet salad dressings and dipping sauces.

- **Certain intoxicating beverages:** Beer, alcoholic wines and sugary mixed drinks.

Though carbs should be limited, low-glycemic fruits such as apples, berries and can be enjoyed in limited quantity as long as you're maintaining a keto-friendly macronutrient series.

Ensure you select healthy food sources and steer clear of processed meals and harmful fats.

The items below should be let alone:

- **Harmful fats:** Margarine, some vegetable oils which are canola and corn oil.

- **Processed meals:** Fast food, canned items, packaged foods and processed meats which can be hot dogs and noon meats.

- **Fast foods:** Meals that include artificial colors, preservatives and sweeteners such as sugary alcohols and aspartame.

Keto-Friendly Brew (Beverage)

Sugar can be seen in a wide variety of beverages including juice, soda, chilled tea and chocolate drinks.

While on a ketogenic diet, concentrated-carb drinks must be avoided just like meals high in carb.

It's an open secret that sugary beverages have been associated with various health issues—from obesity to an increased risk of diabetes.

Luckily, there are numerous tasty, sugar-free drinks to choose from, for those on the keto diet.

Keto-friendly beverages that give healthy living include:

- **Water:** Water is the best option for hydration and should be consumed throughout the day.

- **Sparkling water:** Sparkling water can make a brilliant soda substitute.

- **Unsweetened coffee:** Try intense cream to add flavor to your cup of drink.

- **Unsweetened green tea:** Green tea is everywhere these days, it is appetizing and gives many health benefits.

If you want to include some extra flavor to your drink or water, try different keto-friendly flavor mixtures.

For instance, pitching some fresh mint and lemon peel into your portable water, this can make hydration a breeze.

Though alcohol should be constrained, getting pleasure from a low-carb drink like Vodka, Jack Daniels or Tequila mixed with soda water is a good blend.

DIVERSE TYPES OF FASTING

The usefulness of intermittent fasting (IF) is becoming progressively more well-known amongst those who want to lose weight. From losing obstinate fat and curbing cravings, to lowering inflammation and improving your gut microbiome, intermittent fasting almost seems too good to be true. But not all varieties of fasting are easy—it can be hard to abstain from food for a long time.

So, is there an easier approach to get the benefits of intermittent fasting without going 16-24 hours without a meal or skipping your preferred food of the day?

Diet

Diet is related to the 24-hour fast and the alternate fast in which you will be fasting for 24-hour periods.

But it's faintly easier because you'll only fast twice weekly. It's like this:

- You eat normally for five days weekly.

- You fast completely for two days weekly or peg your intake of calories to 500-600 calories daily on fasting days.

- You can pick when you fast; for instance, dive into one 48-hour fast or fast for two 24-hour periods. Do this as much as you can and be conscious about your health.

This is a little more intense, so you may desire to take advantage of those low-calorie meals while fasting. Just don't surpass 500-600 calories daily to stay in a fasting-mimicking state. And don't forget to stick to healthy fats, protein, and veggies only so you don't experience carb cravings or dramatic reductions in blood sugar.

CHAPTER SEVEN

PHYSICAL EXERCISE IN YOUR ROUTINE

INTERMITTENT FASTING AND

KETOGENIC DIET

If you're undergoing IF or you're fasting for other reasons and you still want to get your exercise in, there are some pros and cons to think of before you decide to work out in a fasted state.

Some studies show that exercising while fasting endangers muscle chemistry and metabolism that's connected to insulin sensitivity and the steady control of the rate of blood sugar. Studies also support eating and immediately engaging in workout before digestion or absorption starts. This is usually helpful to anyone with type 2 diabetes or a metabolic condition.

Undergoing efficient gym sessions while fasting

If you're set to try IF while continuing your exercise routine, there are some things you can do to make your workout helpful.

1. Plan through timing

Christopher Shuff, a registered dietician, says there are three major considerations to make workout more helpful while fasting: he says you can exercise before, during, or after the fueling period.

2. Choose the type of workout based on your macros

It's vital to pay attention to the macronutrients you consume in the day before you exercise and when you eat after. For instance, strength workouts usually require more carbohydrates, while cardio/HIIT [high-intensity interval training] can be done on a lesser carb day.

3. Eat the right foods after your exercise to build or maintain muscle

The most preferred answer for combining IF and exercise is to ensure you exercise during your eating time so your nutrition levels are spiky. "And if you are not doing light lifting, it's crucial for your body to have protein after the (exercise) calisthenics to help with regeneration."

Please note, ensure carbohydrates are eaten after all intense exercise or training and it is wise to have meals that contain not more than 20 grams of protein within 30 minutes after your daily workout.

How can you cautiously exercise while fasting?

The achievement of any weight loss or work out course lies in how safe it is to maintain over time. Staying or camping in a safe location is paramount if you want to maintain your fitness level. More helpful nuggets are outlined below.

Eat reasonable meals while going for high-intensity exercise

This is where a meal calendar comes in. Timing a meal close to a moderate workout is crucial. This way your body has some stored glycogen to fuel your workout.

Be hydrated all the time

Remember, fasting doesn't mean elimination of water. In fact, water is recommended while fasting.

Make sure your electrolytes are up

Coconut aids those that work out to stay hydrated. It stores electrolytes, is low in calories, and tastes really good. Sports drinks are high in sugar, so evade drinking a lot of them.

Keep the intensity and time spent fairly low

If you push yourself too hard and start to feel wobbly or light-headed, take time off. Listening to your body is paramount.

Consider the type of fast that suits you

If you're doing a 24-hour intermittent fast, you should stay with low-intensity exercise such as walking, restorative yoga, or light Pilates. But if you're doing the 16:8 type of fasting, much of the 16-hour fasting window is in the evening, try to sleep, and exercise early in the day. So, the type of workout you do is determined by the kind of fasting you do.

Pay attention to your body

The most important information to heed when exercising during IF is to pay attention to your body. "If you start to feel weak or lightheaded, chances are you're experiencing low blood sugar or you are dehydrated. If that's the case, then go for a carbohydrate-electrolyte drink instantly and then follow up with a well-balanced meal."

While exercising and intermittent fasting usually work for some people, others may not feel relaxed doing any form of exercise while fasting. Check with your doctor or nutritionist before commencing any nutrition or exercise plan.

Get Started with Intermittent Fasting

Intermittent fasting is a program with various formulas, you can try to take advantage of the many proven benefits like: weight loss, disease prevention/treatment, ketosis, improved mental and physical performance and overall wellbeing and fitness.

How much and how fasting results show may vary, and what you do eat during your eating windows should be maximized for your own unique body and daily caloric wants.

If in the past or present, you struggled with a chaotic eating habit, then intermittent fasting is not advisable for you. Fasting may make your situation worse, or trigger it to return. To gain all the benefits, fasting needs to be part of a healthy and balanced diet.

The Truth About Intermittent Fasting

As a Woman, you may have heard of the "moderate" fasting for women called crescendo fasting because most people believe IF benefits men and not women. Hormonal and genetic differences are part of the reasons.

Female Hormones and Intermittent Fasting Women's hormones are more responsive to changes in the environment; this is why many people believe they respond in different ways. For example, it triggers the hunger hormones named leptin and ghrelin.

So what activates hormonal responses?

- Too little meals and poor food choices.
- Too much work out.
- Too much stress, either from too much exercise or from mental strain.
- Too little sleep: Inadequate rest/recovery time.
- Contagion and inflammation (sickness).

None of the above should occur with an IF program carried out excellently.

Debunking Intermittent Fasting Studies for Women

Rats were used for the test. It is often asked scientifically if women should fast, or should fast in a different way. In the test, the rats only ate every other day for 12 weeks. Fourteen days into the study, the female rats' hormones were already out of whack, their monthly periods ended and their ovaries shrunk. Horrible, yes it is.

But it is important to reveal two things to you:

1. Rats live only a few years. One full day's fasting for a rat can be comparable to depriving a human being of food for many days. That's called starvation mode, it would throw your bodily functions off-kilter, and is definitely not advisable for women or men.

2. Calorie constraint during intermittent fasting is not as severe as what the rats were put through.

According to this study, alternate day fasting won't make you lose weight faster than the usual 16/8 method.

So Should Women Do The Crescendo program of Intermittent Fasting?

The crescendo program is similar to 16/8, alternate-day, and the 5/2 fasting program: You should fast for 12-16 hours on non-consecutive days. The assumption behind it, is that it wouldn't "shock" your hormones or raise your appetite.

Another variation is 16/8 turned into 14/10 for ladies. Instead of letting doubt or scientific facts discourage or confound you, the best advice is to pay attention to your body. Everyone is different, man or woman. What worked for your sibling may not work for you, even with the same weight size, height, tribe, exposure and gender.

When you try intermittent fasting, pick a program that suits your body and wellbeing. If you're a breakfast person, your 16/8 program allows you to omit a meal instead of breakfast. If you find 14/10 works better for you, then don't hesitate to go for it. More importantly, ensure you eat enough calories! Consult your doctor or dietician before starting intermittent fasting or the ketogenic diet (or both). Fasting is not advisable for pregnant or nursing mothers, those who are planning to get pregnant or adolescent/pre-adolescent girls.

INTERMITTENT FASTING AND OTHER DIETS

Intermittent fasting isn't an eating regimen, it's an

eating design. Consequently, it bodes well to join intermittent fasting with the eating regimen (or way of life) that suits your necessities.

Look at an Intermittent Fasting Diet Plan.

BEGINNING WITH INTERMITTENT FASTING:

Try not to eat.

Truly. It is that basic. Start by skipping a meal (a great many people pick breakfast or dinner).

Pick a fast style that suits your necessities and way of life.

REMAIN HYDRATED WHILE INTERMITTENT FASTING:

It's significant that you remain hydrated while fasting. Drink water!

Be that as it may, there are two or three different choices of zero-calorie, no sugar (genuine or fake) refreshments you can try.

Water: Yes, I said it—it's the best. You ought to drink mainly water.

Tea: You can drink hot or cold tea. NO SUGAR.

Espresso: Black. NO SUGAR.

You shouldn't have milk or cream while fasting. It will still affect your fast. Be that as it may, if you simply MUST, utilize the smallest amount you can and attempt to gradually wean yourself off of it.

ISN'T BREAKFAST THE MOST IMPORTANT MEAL OF THE DAY? No. That is all.

SPREAD THE RICHES

If you're doing intermittent fasting, you're effectively deciding to skip meals to shed pounds or improve your wellbeing. Be that as it may, there is a large number of individuals everywhere throughout the world who don't consume enough food to meet their absolute minimum day by day health necessities.

There are different techniques for intermittent fasting, and individuals will favor various styles. Here are seven unique approaches to do intermittent fasting.

1. Fast for 12 hours per day

Various styles of intermittent fasting may suit various

individuals. The principles for this eating regimen are basic. An individual needs to settle on and hold fast to a 12-hour fasting window consistently.

As per a few analysts, fasting for 10–16 hours can make the body transform its fat stores into vitality, which discharges ketones into the circulation system. This ought to encourage weight reduction.

This sort of intermittent fasting plan might be a decent alternative for fledglings. This is on the grounds that the fasting window is generally little, a significant part of the fasting happens during rest, and the individual can consume a similar number of calories every day.

The least demanding approach to do the 12-hour fast is to remember the time of rest for the fasting window. For instance, an individual could decide to fast between 7 p.m. and 7 a.m. They would need to complete their meal before 7 p.m. and hold up until 7 a.m. to have breakfast. However, they would be snoozing for a significant part of the time in the middle.

2. Fasting for 16 hours

Fasting for 16 hours every day, leaving an eating window of 8 hours, is known as the 16:8 strategy or the

Leangains diet.

During the 16:8 eating regimen, men fast for 16 hours every day, and ladies fast for 14 hours. This sort of intermittent fast might be useful for somebody who has just attempted the 12-hour fast however didn't perceive any advantages. On this fast, individuals, for the most part, finish their night meal by 8 p.m. and afterward skip breakfast the following day, not eating again until early afternoon.

An investigation on mice found that constraining the eating window to 8 hours shielded them from heftiness, irritation, diabetes, and liver ailment.

Fasting for 2 days every week: Individuals keeping the 5:2 eating routine eat standard measures of empowering food for 5 days and decrease calorie admission on the other 2 days. During the 2 fasting days, men by and large devour 600 calories and ladies 500 calories. Commonly, individuals separate their fasting days in the week. For instance, they may fast on a Monday and Thursday and eat regularly on different days. There ought to be in any event 1 non-fasting day between fasting days.

There is constrained research on the 5:2 eating

regimen, which is otherwise called the Fast eating routine. An investigation including 107 overweight or stout ladies found that confining calories twice week after week and persistent calorie limitation both prompted comparable weight reduction. The investigation likewise found that this eating routine diminished insulin levels and improved insulin affectability among members.

A little scope study took a gander at the impacts of this fasting style in 23 overweight ladies. Through the span of one menstrual cycle, the ladies lost 4.8 percent of their body weight and 8.0 percent of their absolute muscle to fat ratio. Be that as it may, these estimations came back typical for the greater part of the ladies following 5 days of ordinary eating.

3. Alternate day fasting

There are a few varieties of the alternate day fasting plan, which includes fasting every other day.

For certain individuals, alternate day fasting implies a total limitation of strong foods on fasting days, while others permit up to 500 calories. On feeding days, individuals regularly decide to eat as much as they need.

One investigation reports that alternate day fasting is successful for weight reduction and heart wellbeing in both solid and overweight grown-ups. The specialists found that the 32 members lost a normal of 5.2 kilograms (kg), or a little more than 11 pounds (lb), over a 12-week time span.

Alternate day fasting is a serious outrageous type of intermittent fasting, and it may not be reasonable for novices or those with certain ailments. It might likewise be hard to keep up with this kind of fasting in the long haul.

4. A week by week 24-hour fast

On a 24-hour diet, an individual can have teas and no-calorie drinks.

Fasting totally for 1 or 2 days per week, known as the Eat-Stop-Eat diet, includes eating no food for 24 hours one after another. Numerous individuals fast from breakfast to breakfast or lunch to lunch.

Individuals on this eating routine arrangement can have water, tea, and other drinks without calories during the fasting time frame.

Individuals should come back to typical eating designs

on the non-fasting days.

A 24-hour fast can be testing, and it might cause weakness, migraines, or peevishness. Numerous individuals find that these impacts become less extraordinary after some time as the body changes with this new example of eating. Individuals may profit by attempting a 12-hour or 16-hour fast before changing to the 24-hour fast.

5. Meal skipping

This adaptable way to deal with intermittent fasting might be useful for amateurs. It includes infrequently skipping meals. Individuals can choose which meals to avoid according to their degree of yearning or time limitations. Be that as it may, it is imperative to eat empowering foods at every meal.

Meal skipping is probably going to be best when people screen and react to their body's yearning signals. Basically, individuals utilizing this style of intermittent fasting will eat when they are ravenous and skip meals when they are most certainly not. This may feel more normal for certain individuals than the other fasting strategies.

6. The Warrior Diet

The Warrior Diet is a generally extraordinary type of intermittent fasting.

The Warrior Diet includes eating practically nothing, normally only a couple of servings of crude leafy foods, during a 20-hour fasting window, at that point eating one enormous meal around evening time. The eating window is typically just around 4 hours.

This type of fasting might be best for individuals who have attempted different types of intermittent fasting as of now. Supporters of the Warrior Diet guarantee that people are normal nighttime eaters and that eating around evening time permits the body to pick up supplements in accordance with its circadian rhythms.

During the 4-hour eating stage, individuals should ensure that they consume a lot of vegetables, proteins, and fortifying fats. They ought to likewise include a few starches.

In spite of the fact that it is conceivable to eat a few foods during the fasting time frame, it very well may be tasking to adhere to the severe rules on when and what to eat in the long haul. Likewise, a few people battle with eating such an enormous meal so near sleep time.

There is additionally a hazard that individuals on this eating regimen won't eat enough supplements, for example, fiber. This can build the danger of disease and adversely affect digestive wellbeing.

Tips for keeping up intermittent fasting

Yoga and light exercise may assist with making intermittent fasting simpler. It may be difficult to adhere to an intermittent fasting program. The accompanying tips may assist individuals with remaining on target and boost the advantages of intermittent fasting:

Remaining hydrated. Drink loads of water and calorie drinks, for example, home grown teas, for the duration of the day.

Abstaining from focusing on food. Plan a lot of interruptions on fasting days to abstain from pondering on food, for example, making up for lost time with administrative work or heading out to see a film.

Resting and unwinding. Stay away from strenuous

exercises on fasting days, albeit light exercise, for example, yoga might be helpful.

Eating high-volume foods. Select filling yet low-calorie foods, which include popcorn, crude vegetables, and organic products with high water content, for example, grapes and melon.

Expanding taste without calories. Season meals liberally with garlic, herbs, flavors, or vinegar. These foods are incredibly low in calories yet are brimming with taste, which may assist with lessening sentiments of yearning.

Picking supplement-rich foods after the fasting time frame. Eating foods that are high in fiber, nutrients, minerals, and different supplements assists with keeping glucose levels consistent and prevents supplement inadequacies. A fair eating routine will likewise add to weight reduction and wellbeing.

There is a wide range of approaches to do intermittent fasting, and there is no single arrangement that will work for everybody. People will encounter the best outcomes if they evaluate the different styles to perceive what suits their way of life and inclinations.

Regardless of the kind of intermittent fasting, fasting for broadened periods when the body is ill-equipped can be dangerous.

These types of abstaining from excessive food intake may not be reasonable for everybody. If an individual is inclined to scattered eating, these methodologies may worsen their unfortunate relationship with food.

Individuals with wellbeing conditions, including diabetes, ought to consult a specialist before endeavoring any type of fasting.

For the best outcomes, it is basic to eat an energizing and adjusted eating routine on non-fasting days. If essential, an individual can look for proficient assistance to customize an intermittent fasting design and keep away from traps.

Q:

Are a wide range of intermittent fasting styles safe?

A:

Individuals have worked on fasting for a large number of years, however its wellbeing depends more on who is doing the fasting than the style of fasting itself.

Individuals who have malabsorption, are in danger of low glucose, or have other ailments should look for the insight of their health specialist. While the vast majority can practice many fasting styles securely, outrageous sorts of intermittent fasting, for example, the Warrior Diet, can prompt lacking admission of supplements, for example, fiber.

3 DIFFERENT TYPES OF FATS AND THEIR USES EXPLAINED

In the course of the most recent few years, fasting's ubiquity has expanded significantly as terms like intermittent fasting and time-limited eating have advanced into the prevailing press. In any case, before jumping straight into fasting, it's critical to know precisely what fasting is, it's essentials, and the three distinct kinds of fasts.

FASTING EXPLAINED

Fasting is the act of abandoning food for an all-inclusive timeframe. Looking back at our base beginnings, fasting was a part of regular daily existence. During this time it was a test to source for our foods and consequently it was ordinary to abandon food for an all-inclusive timeframe. Fast-forward to the 21st century and sourcing food is never again an issue, in actuality we can have it conveyed to our home at the tap of a button.

With this new period in food sourcing, our washrooms and coolers are bounteous as could be. However simultaneously, fasting has picked up ubiquity and is touted as a 'speedy' hack to achieve your wellness objectives. Be that as it may, fasting isn't for everybody and before you start confining your eating, there are a few essentials to remember.

THE PREREQUISITES OF FASTING

So as to gain the option to fast, there are some basic practices that should first be in place.

Whoever is fasting needs to exhibit healthy living practices which include getting enough rest, getting enough sun, drinking enough water, and eating food altogether (we call these the fundamental way of life rules).

Second, have a quality eating routine and have the option to keep up glucose levels for the duration of the day.

THE BENEFITS OF FASTING:

Mental sharpness: Research and observational proof has indicated that being in a fasted state can improve subjective function. Build and keep up a sound gut: Removing food for a while offers the gut a reprieve from processing and absorbing supplements and can profit the microbiome.

Lower pressure burden and aggravation: Fasting has been shown to bring down irritation by lessening oxidative pressure and has additionally been shown to bring down insulin opposition.

Fasting can be utilized as an instrument for weight reduction, yet is frequently not a practical long term arrangement and can make hazardous practices. For weight reduction, the essentials recorded above are the best arrangement.

FASTING AND FEMALE HORMONES

In the fantastic plan of your life's wellbeing choices, exploring different avenues regarding IF appears to be small, isn't that so? Sadly — for certain ladies, at any rate — it appears as though little choices can have huge effects. Things being what they are, the hormones controlling key capacities like ovulation are unfathomably touchy to your vitality consumption. In

people, hypothalamic-pituitary-gonadal (HPG) hub —
the helpful working of three endocrine organs — acts
somewhat like an air traffic controller.

In the first place, the nerve center discharges
gonadotropin discharging hormone (GnRH). This
advises the pituitary to discharge luteinizing hormone
(LH) and follicular invigorating hormone (FSH). LH and
FSH at that point follow up on the gonads (a.k.a.
testicles or ovaries). In ladies, this triggers the creation
of estrogen and progesterone — which we have to
discharge a developed egg (ovulation) and to form a
pregnancy.

In men, this triggers the creation of testosterone and
sperm. Since this chain of responses occurs on an
unmistakable, ordinary cycle in ladies, GnRH beats
must be absolutely coordinated, or everything can
escape. GnRH beats appear to be delicate to natural
factors, and can be lost by fasting.

Indeed, even transient fasting (state, three days)
modifies hormonal heartbeats in certain ladies.
There's even some proof that missing a solitary
customary meal (while obviously not establishing a
crisis without anyone else) can begin to put us on alert,
livening up our receiving wires so our bodies are
prepared to rapidly react to the adjustment in vitality

consumption if it proceeds.

Perhaps this is the reason certain ladies do fine and dandy with IF while others run into issues. For what reason does IF influence ladies' hormones more than men's? Be that as it may, it may have something to do with kisspeptin, a protein-like atom that neurons use to communicate with one another (and complete significant actions). Kisspeptin animates GnRH creation in both genders, and we realize that it's delicate to leptin, insulin, and ghrelin — hormones that direct and respond to appetite and satiety. Curiously, females have more kisspeptin than males. More kisspeptin neurons may mean more prominent affectability to changes in vitality balance.

This might be one motivation behind why fasting all the more promptly causes ladies' kisspeptin creation to plunge, hurling their GnRH off center.

FERTILITY AND DIGESTION IN RELATION TO WEIGHT LOSS

You may be thinking: So, what's the big deal if kisspeptin drops off and I miss a couple of periods? I'm not having children in the near future, in any case.

The female conceptive framework and digestion are profoundly interlaced. If you're missing periods, you can wager that a lot of hormones have been disturbed—not simply the ones that assist you with getting pregnant. As a rule, ladies will in general eat less protein than men. Fasting ladies, clearly, will consume even less.

Devouring less protein implies taking in less amino acids. Amino acids are expected to enact estrogen receptors and combine insulin-like development factor (IGF-1) in the liver. IGF-1 triggers the uterine divider covering to thicken and the movement of the conceptive cycle.

What's more, critically, estrogen isn't only for proliferation. We have estrogen receptors all through our bodies, remembering for our minds, GI tract, and bones. Change estrogen equalization and you change metabolic capacity all at once: discernment, states of mind, processing, recuperation, protein turnover, bone arrangement, etc.

With regards to hunger and vitality balance, estrogen works in a couple of ways.

To start with, in the brainstem, estrogens adjust the

peptides that signal you to feel full (cholecystokinin) or hungry (ghrelin). In the nerve center, estrogens likewise animate neurons that stop creation of hunger managing peptides. Accomplish something that makes your estrogen drop, and you could wind up feeling much hungrier — and eating significantly more — than you would under ordinary conditions. Estrogens are hence key metabolic controllers.

Yes, estrogens, plural. Since the proportions of the estrogenic metabolites (estriol, estradiol, and estrone) change after some time. Prior to menopause, estradiol is the enormous player. After menopause, it drops, while estrone remains about the same.

The specific jobs of every one of these estrogens remain muddled. However, some hypothesize that a drop in estradiol may trigger an expansion in fat stockpiling. Why? Since fat is utilized to make estradiol.

This may partly clarify why a few ladies think that it's harder to lose fat after menopause. Furthermore, it may fill in as motivation to think about your regenerative wellbeing — regardless of whether you're not centered around making babies.

Indeed, perhaps, developmentally, you shouldn't make

a decent attempt to get that washboard stomach if you're female.

Low-vitality diets can decrease fruitfulness in ladies. Being too lean is a regenerative impediment. Female bodies are stunningly tuned to any dangers to vitality and richness.

At the point when you consider it, this bodes well.

Human females are absolutely interesting in the mammalian world. Get this: Nearly all different vertebrates can end or delay a pregnancy practically at whatever point they have to. You've known this since middle school wellbeing class: Female people can't.

In people, the placenta ruptures the maternal veins, and the hatchling is in complete control.

The infant can obstruct the activity of insulin so as to accumulate more glucose for itself. The baby can even cause the mother's veins to expand, changing the circulatory strain to get tightly to more supplements.

That infant is resolved to survive regardless of the expense to the mother. This wonder, which researchers really contrast with the host-infection relationship, is what's known as "maternal-fetal clash."

When a lady gets pregnant, she can't flatter the embryo to quit developing. The outcome: Fertility at an inappropriate time — like, during a starvation — could be lethal.

The thought was that if your fat store plunged beneath a specific rate (something like 11 percent may be a sensible theory), hormones would fail and your period would stop. Then: no danger of pregnancy.

If there isn't a lot to eat, you'll lose muscle versus fat after some time.

Be that as it may, the circumstance is in reality more complicated than that. All things considered, food accessibility can change rapidly. Furthermore, — as you likely know if you've at any point attempted to get more fit — muscle versus fat regularly requires a significant stretch of time to drop, regardless of whether or not you're eating less calories.

In the interim, ladies who aren't particularly lean can likewise quit ovulating and lose their periods.

That is the reason researchers have come to speculate that general vitality parity might be more critical to this procedure than muscle versus fat ratio as such.

Stressors and vitality balance

In particular, negative vitality balance in ladies might be as a result of the hormonal domino impact we've been discussing. Furthermore, it's not just about how much food you eat.

Negative vitality parity can result from:

- too little food
- poor sustenance
- an excess of activity
- an excess of stress
- sickness, disease, incessant irritation
- too little rest and recuperation

Hell, we can even go through vitality saves by attempting to keep warm.

Any mix of the following stressors could be sufficient to place you into negative vitality parity and stop ovulation: preparing for a long distance race and nursing an influenza; an excessive number of days straight at the rec center and insufficient foods grown from the ground; intermittent fasting and busting your butt to pay the home loan.

You're thinking, did she just reference paying the home

loan? Of course. Mental pressure can completely assume a job in harming our hormonal harmony. Our bodies can't differentiate between a genuine danger and something nonexistent produced by our musings and sentiments. (For example, stressing over how you will get abs.)

The pressure hormone cortisol represses our companion GnRH, and stifles the ovaries' creation of estrogen and progesterone.

In the interim, progesterone is changed over to cortisol during stress, so more cortisol implies less progesterone. This prompts estrogen strength in the HPG pivot. More issues.

You could be floating at 30 percent fat. In any case, if your vitality balance is negative for a long sufficient opportunity, generation stops.

What to do now

In view of what we know, intermittent fasting most likely influences regenerative wellbeing if the body considers it to be a noteworthy stressor.

Anything that influences your conceptive wellbeing influences your general wellbeing and wellness.

Regardless of whether you don't plan to have children.

In any case, intermittent fasting conventions shift, with some being significantly more extraordinary than others. What's more, factors such as your age, healthful status, the time allotment you fast, and different worries throughout your life—including exercise—are additionally likely significant.

So. Is fasting for you?

Taking into account how much stays indistinct, I would recommend a preservationist approach.

If you need to attempt intermittent fasting, start with a delicate convention, and focus on how things are going.

Stop intermittent fasting if:

- your menstrual cycle stops or gets unpredictable
- you have issues nodding off or staying unconscious
- your hair drops out
- you begin to have dry skin or skin inflammation

- you're seeing you don't recuperate from exercises easily
- your wounds are delayed to mend, or you get each bug moving around
- your resistance to stretch reduces
- your dispositions begin swinging
- your heart begins beating in an abnormal manner
- your enthusiasm for pleasure misfires (and your woman parts quit valuing it when it occurs)
- your assimilation eases back down recognizably
- you generally appear to feel cold

Fasting isn't for everybody

In all actuality, a few types of ladies ought not to test trouble.

Try not to attempt intermittent fasting if:

- you're pregnant
- you have a background marked by disarranged eating
- you are incessantly focused
- you don't rest soundly
- you're new to eating less carbs and exercise

Pregnant ladies have additional vitality needs. So if you're beginning a family, fasting is certainly not a smart thought. Likewise if you're under incessant pressure or you aren't resting soundly. Your body needs sustaining, not extra pressure.

What's more, if you've battled with disarranged eating previously, you likely perceive that a fasting convention could lead you down a way that may make further issues for you. Why upset your wellbeing? You can accomplish comparable advantages in different manners. If you're new to slimming down and exercise, IF might resemble an enchantment slug for weight reduction.

Be that as it may, you'd be much more brilliant to address any wholesome inadequacies before you begin trying different things with fasts. Ensure you're beginning from a strong healthful establishment first.

What to do if fasting isn't for you

How might you get in shape if intermittent fasting is certainly not a decent choice for you?

It's basic, really. Get familiar with the fundamentals of good food. It's by a wide margin the best thing you can accomplish for your wellbeing and wellness. Cook and eat entire foods. Exercise consistently. What's more, if you'd like some assistance to do all this, enlist a mentor.

Indeed, intermittent fasting might be mainstream. What's more, perhaps your sibling, your sweetheart or your better half, or even your father thinks that it's a fantastic guide to wellness and wellbeing. Be that as it may, ladies are not quite the same as men, and our bodies have various requirements. Tune in to your body. Furthermore, do what works best for you.

1. Intermittent fasting is simply one more prevailing fashion diet

Intermittent fasting isn't an eating routine by any means. It is a way to deal with eating that calls for halting all food admission (fasting) for at least fourteen hours every day. There are no food limitations, or uncommon food sources to eat a greater amount of, or costly shakes to purchase, or bone soup to consume. You can eat and drink whatever you like, in whatever amount you like. There is no compelling reason to check calories, focuses, carbs, fats, protein, fiber content, macros, micros, or grams of sugar or some other supplement. At an ideal opportunity to eat, you basically make the most of your food until you're fulfilled, then you quit eating for the afternoon.

Presently, if you truly need to check calories, squint at food marks, and so on or you basically love keeping a monotonous diary of each item that passes your lips, IF won't stop you. It's perfect with those methodologies even as it renders them superfluous. In any case, it is anything but an eating routine. It's a way of life.

Is it a trend? For individuals who attempt it for two or three weeks and surrender, sure. Be that as it may, in light of the fact that a few people have gotten on board with a fleeting trend and hopped off doesn't mean intermittent fasting is inadequate.

2. You're starving yourself and destroying your digestion

Accepting you have any put-away fat, consider the possibility that it permits your body to take advantage of it. Dr. Jason Fung focuses on depicting why that is, yet basically, fasting lets your insulin levels drop with the goal that your body can escape fat-stockpiling mode and get into fat-consuming mode, a.k.a. ketosis. When it does this, your digestion doesn't have any motivation to back off. Without random meals, snacks, chewing gum, breath mints, and "diet" drinks, the body can at long last tap into those ample stores.

3. You'll get fantastically Angry!

You switch from being a sugar burner to a fat eliminator by fasting until every one of those glycogen stores are no more. For most people, that implies intermittent fasting a few days straight or undertaking a couple of longer fasts (36–72-hour fasts. Anything longer ought to be done under direct clinical supervision). This gives the body no choice but to begin consuming fat.

You may encounter a "holder" for a couple of days or even half a month, however, it will leave. You can limit early IF holder by gradually developing to longer fasts.

4. Intermittent Fasting is too difficult to even think about sticking with

It's most certainly not. You know what is difficult to stick with? Never again eating frozen yogurt, drinking a brew, getting a charge out of a pizza, a taco, or having oats chocolate chip treats hot out of the broiler.

The magnificence of IF is you can eat anything you desire, which means treats lose their "gorge" request and blame affectation since they aren't ever beyond reach. Even under the least favorable conditions, they're postponed for a couple of hours.

The key for some individuals isn't bouncing in attempting to do 24-hour fasts immediately. Beginning little, at 16 hours or even less, and step by step stirring your way up to longer fasts can make this way of life much simpler in the first place and easier to stick to.

5. Fasting "deceives the body" into eating less calories

"Calories in/calories out" is the genuine weight reduction fantasy. You can never surpass your fork.

6. There are things you can eat while fasting

Bone juices have no part in a viable fast. Neither bulletproof espresso, diet pop, chewing gum, nuts, celery sticks, or sticky nutrients. Would you be able to eat those things? Sure. Is it fasting? No! Simply stop. Quit stuffing food into your face since that is not fasting. Fasting will be fasting. That is the general purpose.

Do you love bone juices? Fantastic. Make them during your eating window. Can't survive without your impenetrable espresso? Put it in your window. Love sound, low-carb nuts? Eat them in your window. Dependent on Diet Coke or natural product seasoned LaCroix? Window, window, window. That is the point at which you can eat anything you desire and enjoy sweet and fruity drinks, vodka, or whatever makes your day.

Gin Stephens, creator of Delay Don't Deny, calls her methodology "clean fasting." It takes into account plain water, shimmering water, plain dark or decaf espresso (no frou-frou enhanced espressos but natural product seasoned waters) and plain dark or decaf tea (no sweet or fruity herbals). The splendid thing about this methodology is that when you tail it, you're less ravenous than you'd be if animating your craving with every one of these things columnists (who haven't really attempted or prevailed at IF in the long term) need you to believe is "fine" to have while "fasting."

Possibly, writers and bloggers make these cases about "what's OK to stuff in your face while fasting" since that is the thing that individuals need to hear. They need to hear that they can "fast" while eating and never experience a solitary craving for food. Notwithstanding what we might need to hear, that is not what works.

The incongruity is that these things we're being advised "it's OK to eat while fasting" (what an ironic expression that is!) invigorate hunger and make "fasting" a whole lot harder.

Gin shed 80 pounds with her way to deal with IF and has kept it off for a long time by getting a charge out of one huge, solid meal in a window of around four hours out of each day.

7. Be that as it may, however yet keto, however! Fats don't raise glucose, so overwhelming whipping cream and avocados and nuts are fine to have while fasting, isn't that so?

Once more, no. Such a large number of individuals are conflating foods that don't expand blood glucose with things that do invigorate insulin. If it's food, it will invigorate insulin. If it's enhanced, particularly if it's sweet, it might expand your insulin (everybody is unique) so why risk it? Insulin is a clever hormone that switches your body over to fat stockpiling mode. To consume fat, you must let your insulin descend and allow your body to get to those fat stores for vitality. This is the thing that the F (fasting) part of IF does.

Regardless of whether a few foods don't invigorate insulin and intrude on ketosis (and I figure they do, yet how about we not sit around idly contending that point), your body is still going to need to consume off the fat in that hot buttered espresso or avocado or a bunch of pecans before it will try taking advantage of your put-away fat. So if you're here to lose fat or are battling with incredible craving during your fast, in any event attempt clean fasting before surrendering.

8. It's difficult to get all the calories and additionally supplements you need in a short eating window.

9. You'll restore everything when you stop

While in fact this might be valid, it's valid for each weight reduction approach in the world. Stop your keto diet, what occurs? Stop Weight Watchers and watch your scale creep back up. Come back to your old eating designs following quite a while of Shakeology and hit me up on to what extent those new thin pants fit. As Gin Stephens likes to call attention to, all weight control plans work when you stick to them and "fall flat" when you stop.

Yet, since it is anything but an eating regimen, IF offers three unmistakable favorable circumstances long after you stop.

It will in general control your hunger so you want less shoddy food and lower food amounts by and large. When you're eating for a time of just a couple of hours every day, you will in general be pickier and the limit of your stomach bit by bit contracts.

It jams digestion and even lifts it. This is on the grounds that once your body takes advantage of its fat stores there is no requirement for it to back your digestion off (as it does with low-calorie abstains from food). Low-calorie abstains from food brief the body to lessen digestion to coordinate the decreased vitality consumption. On IF, the body doesn't have to do that since it's ready to take advantage of put-away fat.

When you've encountered the wonderful vitality and mental clearness of fat-consuming mode, you understand how bad you felt when you were stuffing your face and processing food throughout the day. So regardless of whether you're never again doing intermittent fasting as such, you may wind up eating less regularly at any rate.

The possibility that you're going to stop has a place with the universe of diets, not intermittent fasting. It is a way of life. It is successful, adaptable, supportable, and free. There is no compelling reason to stop, and there is definitely no craving to stop.

10. Intermittent fasting is a celebrated dietary issue

It doesn't take a virtuoso to perceive that somebody who has experienced dietary issues ought to keep away from a way to deal with food that may trigger them to come back to a risky fixation.

In like manner, IF isn't the best methodology for everybody. Individuals with certain wellbeing conditions, on drugs that must be taken with food, youngsters, any individual who is pregnant or nursing should find an alternate methodology. It's constantly a smart thought to consult your primary care physician before rolling out significant improvements to your eating designs.

In any case, none of this makes intermittent fasting a dietary issue. It is basically an example of eating that interchanges brief times of swearing off food with brief times of eating food all the time.

Concentrating on things other than food the entire day and afterward getting a charge out of an energizing and fulfilling meal feels like the sanest way to deal with food.

There are numerous basic confusions with respect to intermittent fasting, how about we attempt to expose some of those legends here.

If you need to check out intermittent fasting but are stressed over some of the things you've heard, it's smarter to adhere to realities.

1) "Your body will enter starvation mode"

Basic idea directs that, if you skip meals, your body goes into starvation mode and begins to slow your digestion, imagining that it is a "period of starvation". This has been the mainstream line of reasoning for quite a while, yet it's really a myth.

Ongoing exploration recommends that you need to not eat for nearly three entire days before your body even begins to bring down your resting metabolic rate. In all actuality, the human body was intended to withstand the impacts of fasting since the time we were stone age men.

Starvation is the point at which your muscle to fat ratio's stores are devoured completely, so it must choose the option to separate muscle for vitality. This won't occur on the grounds that you skipped breakfast.

With intermittent fasting, your body discharges put-away fat and uses it as vitality, while your slender muscle tissue stays immaculate. This is particularly valid if you have a great deal of fat stores effectively, which means your body has a ton to work with.

Late investigations on intermittent fasting likewise propose that fasting is valuable to general wellbeing. Tests done on animals that ate a rich eating regimen of greasy foods in an eight-hour eating window and afterward fasted for the remainder of the day indicated that they didn't get large or show high insulin levels.

2) "You can eat all you need in your eating window"

This is perhaps the greatest legend encompassing intermittent fasting, and accordingly probably the greatest trap for individuals who attempt intermittent fasting and battle with making it work. Because you've fasted for a specific measure of time and are currently in your eating window, doesn't mean you can eat anything you desire.

Getting in shape, even on intermittent fasting, is still

about caloric shortfall. It is extremely unlikely you will get more fit if you surpass your support calories.

Depending on your age, height, weight, and muscle to fat ratio, there is a sure number of calories your body consumes for the duration of the day simply keeping up your present weight. If you eat more than that number of calories during your eating window, at that point you're going to put on weight regardless of to what extent you've fasted.

To keep yourself from indulging, it is ideal to screen your caloric admission. Besides, endeavor to eat a reasonable eating regimen that includes a great deal of foods grown from the ground, and bunches of fiber. Stay away from processed foods and food sources that have a great deal of additives. Stick to crisp, nutritious, and healthy food that is useful for your body.

3) "You'll be constantly hungry"

Perhaps the greatest thing individuals stress over with intermittent fasting is that they could be constantly hungry. It is a startling idea to not have the option to eat for 16 to 18 hours, or even as long as 20 hours every day. Individuals stress that they will be hungry basically consistently until they break their fast, which is a complete and all out legend.

Honestly, there is a "becoming accustomed to" period for intermittent fasting. Before all else, you will encounter cravings for food that make you question what you're doing with your life. Be that as it may, when your body acclimates to its new vitality utilization worldview, it will make changes to the manner in which your body works — including sentiments of yearning.

Intermittent fasting progressively gets simpler as you slip yourself into it. Start by fasting for 14 hours every day for the initial two weeks, at that point knock your fasting window to 16 hours, until you're prepared for 18 (or remain at 16 hours if that works better for you). Keep in mind, tune in to your body and what it's attempting to let you know. You'll realize when you're prepared to kick it up a score.

4) "It's an enchantment stunt"

While it might unquestionably feel like enchantment, given the speedy and unmistakable advantages, intermittent fasting is upheld by science and numerous examinations have been done throughout the years to investigate its motivation and impacts. In opposition to mainstream thinking, intermittent fasting isn't new. It's been around for a considerable length of time.

Generally, its study is extremely straightforward — exhaust a larger number of calories than you are consuming, and your body will be in a condition of caloric shortfall. This will without a doubt cause weight reduction. Since 3,500 calories make up a pound, cutting 500 calories off your basal metabolic rate every day will guarantee you lose at any rate one pound of weight securely every week.

What intermittent fasting likewise does is it diminishes insulin levels during the fasting time frame, which assists with encouraging fat consumption.

In truth, intermittent fasting takes into consideration increasingly adaptable dietary patterns, which means you can eat a greater amount of the food you appreciate as opposed to eating dull, bland, "solid" food. In any case, don't try too hard. Stick to great, nutritious food yet additionally, don't be reluctant to have a cut of cake now and again.

When You Should Avoid Intermittent Fasting

Intermittent fasting is incredible for certain individuals,

yet for other people, it could be risky. For certain individuals, intermittent fasting (IF) is a finished distinct advantage. It's the way to everything from maintainable weight reduction to expanded mental clearness to a genuine lift in vitality.

In any case, on the grounds that intermittent fasting is the go-to way of life for certain individuals doesn't imply that it's for everybody. While intermittent fasting is a solid decision for a few, for other people, it can really be perilous.

Be that as it may, who precisely ought to maintain a strategic distance from intermittent fasting? What are a portion of the perils? What's more, what are a few choices for individuals who aren't an ideal choice for intermittent fasting—yet at the same time need to receive comparative rewards?

Insulin-Dependent Diabetics

One populace that could put themselves at genuine hazard by following an intermittent fasting plan? Individuals who battle with Type 1 or insulin-subordinate diabetes.

"Intermittent fasting cycles between times of fasting

and unhindered eating. In individuals living with diabetes and who take against diabetic meds, particularly insulin, this could be exceptionally hazardous," says Dr. Rocio Salas-Whalen, endocrinologist and organizer of New York Endocrinology.

"Against diabetic prescriptions, explicitly insulin, will keep on affecting glucose on the fasting days. This could drop sugar levels to a hazardous point," she includes.

Diabetics need to keep up stable glucose levels to remain sound (through both eating regimen and exercise). This can be almost unthinkable with intermittent fasting.

Notwithstanding a solid eating routine, practice is additionally significant.

Continuance Athletes

Preparing for a long-distance race or an up and coming Ironman? If this is true, intermittent fasting likely isn't for you.

"Supplement timing is critical for sports execution and would be a test while following an intermittent fasting diet," says Allison Knott, MS, RDN, CSSD, a New York City-based enlisted dietitian.

"Perseverance sports require expanded calorie needs in light of the overabundance of calories consumed. Also, the effect [that] perseverance practice has on supplement needs previously, during, and after an occasion or long instructional course requires reliable calorie consumption and sufficient macronutrient admission to fix muscle, recharge glycogen stores, and keep up electrolyte balance."

Intermittent fasting doesn't give you the consistent portion of calories and supplements you have to prepare, perform, and recoup. In this way, if you have a perseverance occasion coming up, you should plan to keep away from intermittent fasting. (Follow a more perseverance-friendlyeating arrangement).

Individuals With a History of Disordered Eating

If you're recuperating from scattered eating practices, intermittent fasting is a no-go area. "A few people who will need to dodge intermittent fasting include those with a propensity to confused eating or a background marked by a dietary issue," says Knott.

Intermittent fasting requires times of limitation followed by times of eating bigger meals. This can be very activating for individuals who battle with limiting, gorging, or other disarranged eating designs. In such cases, it's smarter to maintain a strategic distance from intermittent fasting out and out and adhere to a progressively reliable food plan.

Should Pregnant Women Fast?

When you're carrying a child, you have to follow a pregnancy diet that is loaded up with supplements (and calories!) to keep you and your child healthy. Unfortunately, you won't get that with intermittent fasting.

"Individuals with incessant conditions, for example, diabetes or malignant growth, would not have any desire to practice intermittent fasting in view of the potential for low glucose, insufficient calorie admission, and the chance of not meeting sufficient supplement needs. The equivalent is valid for ladies who are pregnant and breastfeeding on account of expanded calorie and supplement needs," says Knott.

If you're pregnant, you have to eat regularly and enough to help you and your infant's wellbeing. The structure of intermittent fasting simply doesn't take that into account.

Are there options in contrast to intermittent fasting?

Unmistakably, intermittent fasting isn't for everybody. In any case, if the intermittent fasting way of life isn't for you, is there an approach to receive all the rewards of intermittent fasting (like weight reduction, expanded vitality, ideal fat consuming, and better fixation) without putting yourself in danger?

The appropriate response is yes—with a pledge to a sound, even way of life. Also, while that arrangement probably won't be as buzz commendable as intermittent fasting, it can surely be similarly as powerful.

"Quite a bit of what we think about food doesn't have feature-making claim since it's exhausting. Eat more plants, pick heart sound fats, eat lean animal proteins (if you need)— yet additionally include plant proteins—center around assortment, drink water, maintain a strategic distance from included sugars, limit ultra-prepared foods. We all know these things," says Knott. "The key is to make that method for gobbling one that makes up most of your eating routine, most of the time, and for most of your life."

If you have a condition that keeps you from bouncing on board the intermittent fasting train, you can still appreciate all the wellbeing boosting benefits. Roll out positive improvements to your eating routine that you can focus on continuing in the long haul.

You will doubtlessly feel tired due to the fact that your body is running on less vitality than expected, and since fasting can help feelings of anxiety, it can likewise upset your rest designs.

A similar organic chemistry that controls disposition likewise directs craving with supplement utilization influencing the action of synapses like dopamine and serotonin, which assume a role in uneasiness and sadness.

That implies deregulating your hunger may do likewise to your disposition and in this way you will no doubt feel bad tempered whenever you are fasting.

The last recommendation for people who are keen on an intermittent fasting diet is that it restrains your liquor admission just during eating periods. Try not to drink liquor during or following fasting and regardless of whether you drink during your eating periods, remember that drinking liquor implies that you are dislodging your chance for sufficient sustenance.

Fasting and Exercise

In spite of the fact that individuals fast for various reasons, fasting and exercise are regularly embraced together. Depending upon the sort of fast and exercise you complete, it might be a smart idea to consolidate the two—there are various complexities to consider given the various kinds of fasts and physical action that can be matched up. Here are some top-level contemplations around joining physical movement when you're limiting calories.

Individual Health

Research differs on the advantages of exercising while at the same time fasting, as studies are regularly done on generally veering populaces (individuals with metabolic disorder versus continuance competitors, for instance). In any case, a recent report proposes that "long term exercise in the fasted state in sound subjects is related to more noteworthy enhancements in insulin affectability, basal muscle fat take-up limit, and oxidation."

The key takeaway there is "in sound subjects." If you have any wellbeing conditions, you need to make certain to counsel with a clinical expert before you attempt either fasting or exercising to realize which structures are ideal for you.

Timing of Exercise

There are various kinds of fasts, yet one of the most famous structures is the 16:8 intermittent fast (IF), where individuals confine their calorie admission to a 8-hour window, regularly fasting medium-term and frequently skipping breakfast, typically for a delayed timeframe or a few days per week.

Enlisted dietitian Christopher Shuff revealed to Healthline that generally, keeping up run of the mill practice with IF isn't typically an issue. The question is, which window of time will make the exercise the best: previously, during, or after the eating window?

"Working out before the window is perfect for somebody who performs well during exercise on an unfilled stomach, while during the window is more qualified for somebody who doesn't prefer to practice on an empty stomach and furthermore needs to profit by post-exercise sustenance," he said.

When you fast for longer than roughly 14–16 hours, depending upon your metabolic status before starting your fast, your body inevitably utilizes your put-away carbs, or glycogen, as fuel. If you're a fat-adjusted individual, eating a ketogenic diet, you'll travel through the metabolic stages a lot faster than if you are eating an eating regimen inverse to a keto diet (HCLF) as well as if you're not as metabolically adaptable. Some examination recommends that exercising in a fasted state could mean you'll consume more fat than if you've eaten not long previously. Be that as it may, definitive research is restricted, so you might need to attempt an assortment of approaches to perceive how you feel and what results you notice dependent on your objectives.

CHAPTER EIGHT

WHY YOU SHOULD AVOID

INTERMITTENT FASTING

We can also use this means to compare intermittent fasting with keto, shall we? Unlike keto, intermittent fasting can't be classified as a diet. It's an eating method styled around certain feeding and fasting periods which is not helpful to the health of some people. One of the most popular forms of intermittent fasting is the usual 16:8 split, the devotee of this method fasts for 16 hours and only eats during an eight-hour break. It simply means no eating once it is 8 p.m., have time to sleep or take a nap, then have lunch like a king at noon the following day. Other devotees of intermittent fasting might prefer to do an 18:6 split or fast 24 hours every other day.

Intermittent fasting can take many forms and has many opportunities. Like keto, people have used it to shed weight, regulate blood sugar levels, and gain more clarity. When you're fasting, the body doesn't have to discharge insulin to cut body sugar, but it chooses to turn fats into ketones. The best way to know you're improving is if you are not adding fat during your feeding window, you're indeed eating less calories without having to track it. Some people also use intermittent fasting mainly to give their digestive systems a chance to reorganize.

According to Mancinelli, a keto coach for those in the U.S. and the Western world, "the fact is the period of time that we're not eating is so short that your body never gets the chance to use any stored fat. He further said that most Americans don't go for six hours without eating."

Some nutritionists do not believe intermittent fasting is a new style, they believe it is an eating pattern that has been practiced for centuries. Their argument is, over the years, humans have lived through periods of surplus and famine, while many tribes around the globe have something about their forefathers fasting in their history books.

No matter how old and popular fasting is, many people can't spend a day without consuming a meal or else, they will feel lethargic or dizzy. Perfectly healthy adults can go a few days without eating and be absolutely fine. Lots of people believe they can't go a day without eating, though majority haven't tried this.

Are there Opportunities in practicing both keto and intermittent fasting?

Experience has shown that using the ketogenic diet and intermittent fasting will moderate the time one spends in ketosis. This could translate to more weight loss, reduced hunger pangs, and plenty of energy.

Nutritionists also believe it's easier for someone to start a ketogenic diet compared to intermittent fasting. On the other hand, some people believe eating a specified variety of food is difficult, especially if the food you are told to stop eating is your best staple. Another belief is that intermittent fasting makes you go hungry for a long time.

However, every good thing requires a price that must be paid but combining these two methods helps to increase results. Please note that these methods of eating are not for everyone, if you can't sacrifice your appetite or your health does not allow you, it will be great not to try any of these.

What are the risks involved in engaging in both keto and intermittent fasting?

Harley Pasternak, a renowned celebrity trainer and nutritionist specialist, said he would never advise either eating patterns, let alone do them altogether at once.

In his words, he said "I can't talk for anyone who would want to do the two at once, but I personally would not," he emphasized. "It sounds like an excessively regimented, controlled, and antisocial way to survive."

Intermittent fasting and keto might be hard to sustain especially when you're out with associates for a meal or celebrating the holidays with friends. You might be tempted to devour something that you "shouldn't" eat or eat outside of your feeding window. And if you slip, you might be hard on yourself. For many, keto and intermittent fasting might not be doable.

There are even some demerits if you were to observe either eating style separately. For example, sometimes newbie-dieters complain of getting "the keto flu" throughout their transition, which can result in nausea, headaches, faintness and stomach pain. A low-carbohydrate dieter can also be at risk of not providing sufficient vitamins and nutrients like magnesium, potassium, nutrients, calcium, and fiber.

It is an open secret that the healthiest, oldest living populations in the universe are people that tend to eat all classes of food.

Some nutritionists agreed that combining keto and

fasting might be entirely unnecessary because they are not guaranteed of weight loss or fitness. They further said it is not necessarily needed to follow either eating pattern till the end of one's life—especially keto. Remember it is important to be "metabolically flexible at all times."

Another aspect is, it is not advisable medically to lose the capability to use glucose for energy. This is because when you eat something that's glucose rich, your blood sugar is going to be fairly high since you're going to have to develop the mechanisms to use for energy gain due to the previous loss as you're taking less carbohydrates. It is not right to be undergoing ketosis forever. It should be stopped at a point if you're using it as a means to treat some diseases.

Who are those that should not try both?

The combination of intermittent fasting and the ketogenic diet are principally risky for certain types of people.

Children who are not up to the age of 18, who are still developing, for example, should be left to eat whenever they feel like it. Those who have surpassed the age of 65 may have trouble getting adequate nutrients and calories to maintain certain body tissues and body mass, they should avoid any controlled eating rule.

This can also be true for anyone who has a nutritional deficit or for someone who needs to take medication with food. "It's not that you can't do intermittent fasting but you need to be ready medically before you start."

Pregnant women who plan on breastfeeding after giving birth, might not want to delve into intermittent keto fasting to shed the baby weight. Producing milk needs a lot of energy and so controlling calories might not be the best move.

And if you've suffered or are currently suffering from any eating disorders, starting these two eating styles can be very emotionally triggering. It might be paramount to find other means to reach your health aspirations.

What should I do if I'm ready to do keto and intermittent fasting together?

Always seek advice from your doctor or registered nutritionist/dietician before changing up your eating routine. You want to have a solid game plan and know that you are doing it in a way that's healthy for you.

If you've got the permission and don't know where to begin, the calm route is to give intermittent fasting a try first before going the keto route.

"What I advise is trying something that is going to fit into your timetable, don't concentrate on what's the best possible number of hours that you should be fasting, but do what works in your life. Do an account of when you eat and which meals are super essential to you and ask yourself, 'Which one could I take out?' It might not be easy but it is achievable."

After all these, you can try to start keto if you want and see how it goes. Moreover, consult your health expert and find a group of people that can inspire you to stay on track always.

Whatever you decide to do, you have to persist by asking yourself, "What do I think will be sustainable for my way of life?" and "Which eating technique is the best for me?"—don't take note of the physical aspect alone, the mental and emotional areas are also essential.

If you admire the keto diet and like the results, but you can't help but marvel if you can give your weight loss even more of an increase by trying another interesting diet regimen in tandem—then intermittent fasting (IF) is readily available for you. IF is simply a weight loss plan in which you stop eating for periods of time—on swap days (for example). You will need to start scheduling all your meals timetable into a daily time window—like, 8 a.m. to 4p.m., or carefully spread between 9 a.m. and 9 p.m. (It can also be known as the OMAD diet, or "one meal a day.") The question is, is the blend of keto and intermittent fasting safe for everyone?

According to the Academy of Nutrition and Dietetics, the most vital thing is to make sure you're meeting your dietary needs. This means working with a medical/nutrition group. How exactly does an IF-keto regimen continue getting good advice—and what are IF's honest benefits? See the details below.

How the keto diet and intermittent fasting work independently

If you don't know the principles of keto diet, here's what you need to be familiar with. "The ketogenic diet is very low in carb—carbs are limited to 40-60 grams daily, and more than 80% of your calories are gotten from fat. Keto is a modest protein diet—it's intended to force the body into a fat-burning state called 'ketosis'. Ketosis uses an energy supply called ketone bodies to stimulate the brain. So your body is forced to cut fat rather than spending glucose, or blood sugar, for fuel. When the glucose in your body is exhausted, ketone bodies are created. Then, those ketone bodies cross your veins/brain barrier as energy for your brain and (CNS) central nervous system."

Despite the fact that researchers are as yet inquiring about precisely how ketosis influences the body, a few examinations recommend keto diets can:

- Improve state of mind and mental clearness
- Improve heart wellbeing
- Abatement seizures among epilepsy patients
- Help in malignancy medicines (possibly)
- Decline skin break out
- Cutting carbs is a certain method to place your body in a condition of ketosis. Another way? Fasting.

Studies propose intermittent fasting can:

- Increase life span in animals and people
- Increase levels of the human development hormone, advancing solid muscle development and fat loss

- Improve assurance against cardiovascular sicknesses
- Delicately stress your cells and neurons, reinforcing them
- Advance autophagy — a characteristic procedure where cells shed harmed cells, poisons

One especially fascinating advantage of intermittent fasting is that it is by all accounts successful at expanding insulin affectability, which refers to how cells react to insulin—the hormone that advises cells to permit sugar to enter so it tends to be utilized as fuel.

"The food we eat is separated by catalysts in our gut and in the long run winds up as atoms in our circulatory system," Monique Tello, MD, MPH, composed for Harvard Health Blog. "Starches, especially sugars and refined grains (think white flours and rice), are immediately separated into sugar, which our cells use for vitality. If our cells don't utilize everything, we store it in our fat cells as, well, fat. Be that as it may, sugar can just enter our cells with insulin, a hormone made in the pancreas. Insulin carries sugar into the fat cells and keeps it there."

In any case, for reasons researchers don't totally

comprehend, our cells can get impervious to insulin, which can make your pancreas produce a lot of the hormone and afterward, after it gets exhausted, insufficient. Intermittent fasting may break that cycle by placing your body in a fasting state in which it doesn't overproduce insulin, as Dr. Jason Fung told the Bulletproof Radio digital recording:

"If you become very insulin safe, at that point your insulin levels are up constantly, your body is continually attempting to push the vitality into the fat cells, and afterward you feel cold, worn out and lousy. That is the genuine issue. Opposition truly relies upon two things. It's not just the significant levels, but it's also the industriousness of those levels. What individuals have acknowledged is that the insulin obstruction, since it relies upon those two things, a timeframe where you can get your insulin levels exceptionally low is going to break that opposition since it breaks that perseverance. Not just the levels, however, the constancy of those levels."

Combining the keto diet with intermittent fasting

The significant connection between the keto diet and intermittent fasting is that the two of them can place the body into ketosis, by and large bringing about lower levels of glucose and insulin, and along these lines weight reduction. In any case, would they say they are safe to do together?

Intermittent fasting will most likely assist you with arriving at ketosis faster than a keto diet will alone, normally within 24 hours to three days. It's safe to say that, as far as weight reduction is concerned, joining these two methodologies is probably going to improve the other's adequacy. However, saying this doesn't imply that everybody ought to do it.

Intermittent fasting and keto diet carbs have been connected to state of mind issues in the first weeks of starting either fractiousness, uneasiness, burdensome indications. (For keto abstaining from food, this is regularly called the "Keto Influence"). It may be obvious that an uncommon change in dietary propensities would bring about emotional episodes, and, certainly, recounted reports propose these side effects will in general clear up in the long run if individuals adhere to their new schedules.

If you're going to push ahead with combining intermittent fasting with the keto diet, consider these bits of exhortation from Perfect Keto:

"Ensure you, despite everything, eat enough. Intermittent fasting helps you normally eat less during the day, yet be certain you're still eating nutritious ketogenic foods to maintain a strategic distance from any inadequacies or metabolic issues. Utilize a site or application to compute perfect caloric admission and your ketogenic macros for every day, then track them to ensure you're getting adequate sustenance.

Measure your ketone levels. Despite the fact that fasting can truly assist you with remaining in ketosis, it's as yet imperative to ensure you aren't eating such a large number of carbs or doing whatever else to show you out of ketosis. Track your ketones frequently to ensure you're entirely in ketosis!"

CHAPTER NINE

RECIPES

"There are no determinations or limitations about what type or how much food to eat while following intermittent fasting," says Lauren Harris-Pincus, MS, RDN, creator of The Protein-Packed Breakfast Club. In any case, "the advantages [of IF] are not prone to go with predictable meals of Big Macs," says Mary Purdy, MS, RDN, seat of Dietitians in Integrative and Functional Medicine.

Both Pincus and Purdy concur that an even eating routine is the way to getting in shape, keeping up vitality levels, and staying with the eating routine. "Anybody endeavoring to get thinner should concentrate on supplement-rich foods, similar to natural products, veggies, entire grains, nuts, beans, seeds, dairy and fit proteins," Pincus says.

Purdy includes, "My proposals wouldn't be altogether different from foods that I may regularly recommend for improved wellbeing—high-fiber, natural, entire food sources that offer assortment and flavor."

At the end of the day, eat a lot of the following foods and you won't end up in a hungry rage while fasting.

1. Water

Despite the fact that you aren't eating, it's critical to remain hydrated for such a large number of reasons, including the soundness of fundamentally every significant organ in your body. The measure of water that any one individual should drink fluctuates, however, you need your pee to be a light yellow shade consistently. Dull yellow pee demonstrates lack of hydration, which can cause cerebral pains, weakness, and discombobulation. Couple that with constrained food, and it could be a recipe for disaster. If the idea of plain water doesn't energize you, include a crush of lemon squeeze, a couple of mint leaves, or cucumber cuts to your water. It'll be your little mystery.

2. Avocado

It might appear to be irrational to eat the most unhealthy organic product while attempting to shed pounds, yet the monounsaturated fat in avocado is amazingly satisfying. An investigation even found that adding a portion of an avocado to your lunch may keep you full for a considerable length of time longer than if you didn't eat the green diamond.

3. Fish

There's an explanation the Dietary Guidelines proposes: eating, at any rate, eight ounces of fish for each week. In addition to the fact that it is rich in solid fats and protein, it likewise contains plentiful measures of nutrient D. Also, if you're just eating a restricted measure of food for the duration of the day, don't you need one that conveys progressively supplement value for your money? Also, restricting your calorie admission may disturb your discernment, and fish is frequently viewed as a "cerebrum food."

4. Cruciferous Veggies

Foods like broccoli, Brussels sprouts, and cauliflower are on the whole loaded with the f-word—fiber. When you're eating whimsically, it's essential to eat fiber-rich foods that will keep you normal and prevent stoppage. Fiber additionally can cause you to feel full, which is something you may need if you can't eat again for 16 hours.

5. Potatoes

Repeat after me: Not every single white food is awful. A valid example: Studies have seen potatoes as one of the most satisfying foods around. Another examination found that eating potatoes as a major aspect of a sound eating routine could help with weight reduction. Apologies, French fries and potato chips don't tally.

6. Beans and Legumes

Your preferred bean stew might be your closest companion on the IF way of life. Food, especially carbs, supplies vitality for movement. While we're not instructing you to carbo-load, it unquestionably wouldn't hurt to toss some low-calorie carbs, similar to beans and vegetables, into your eating plan. In addition, foods like chickpeas, dark beans, peas, and lentils have been shown to diminish body weight, even without calorie limitation.

7. Probiotics

You know what the little critters in your gut like the most? Consistency and assorted variety. That implies they are unsettled when they're eager. Also, when your gut is distraught, you may encounter some aggravating reactions, similar to blockage. To neutralize this obnoxiousness, include probiotic-rich foods, such as kefir, fermented tea or kraut, to your eating regimen.

8. Berries

Strawberries are an extraordinary wellspring of

immune boosting nutrient C, with an excess of 100 percent of the everyday esteem in one cup. Furthermore, that is not by any means the best section—an ongoing report found that individuals who consumed an eating regimen rich in flavonoids, similar to those in blueberries and strawberries, had littler increments in BMI over a 14-year time frame than the individuals who didn't eat berries.

9. Eggs

One enormous egg has six grams of protein and concocts in minutes. Getting as much protein as could be expected is significant for remaining full and building muscle. One examination found that men who had an egg breakfast rather than a bagel were less ravenous and ate less for the duration of the day. So, when you're searching for something to do during your fasting period, why not hard-heat up some eggs?

10. Nuts

They might be higher in calories than numerous snacks, however nuts contain something that most shoddy foods don't include: the nutrients.

What's more, if you're stressed over calories, don't be!

A recent report found that a one-ounce serving of almonds (around 23 nuts) has 20 percent less calories than recorded on the mark. Fundamentally, the chewing procedure doesn't totally separate the almond cell dividers, leaving a bit of the nut flawless and unabsorbed during processing.

11. Entire Grains

Being on a careful nutritional plan and eating carbs appear as though they have a place in two unique basins, however not generally! Entire grains are rich in fiber and protein, so eating a little goes a long way in keeping you full. Also, another investigation recommends that eating entire grains rather than refined grains may really fire up your digestion. So feel free to eat your entire grains and venture out of your customary range of familiarity to attempt farro, bulgur, spelt, kamut, amaranth, millet, sorghum, or freekeh.

While fasting can be overpowering, particularly if you haven't done it before, intermittent fasting can be significantly simpler than numerous different kinds of eating plans.

When you start your intermittent fasting venture, you'll in all likelihood find that you feel full more and can keep the meals you do eat basic. There are a couple of various ways you can fast, so I separated every one of the various plans below into apprentice, intermediate, and progressed alongside a regular meal plan for every day.

The blend of supplements will give you the vitality you need to upgrade the advantages of your fasting venture. Simply make a point to consider any individual food intolerance, and utilize this as a guide for your specific wellbeing case, and alter from that point.

Keep in mind, intermittent fasting doesn't really mean calorie-controlled, so make certain to eat as indicated by your own caloric needs.

1. The essential intermittent fasting meal plan for novices.

If you are a fledgling, start by just eating between the long periods of 8 a.m. and 6 p.m. This is an incredible method to plunge your toes into the fasting waters. This arrangement permits you to eat each meal in addition to certain bites yet at the same time get in 14 hours of fasting inside a 24-hour duration.

Breakfast: Green Smoothie at 8 a.m. Subsequent to fasting, you can slide into your day of eating with a smoothie since it is somewhat simpler for the gut to process. You'll need to go for a green smoothie rather than a high-sugar natural product smoothie to abstain from beginning your day on a glucose thrill ride. Include loads of sound fats to prop you up until lunch!

Grass-fed liver burgers are one of the best decisions for lunch during the week, and they are amazingly simple to prepare to have all through the whole week. You can eat this on a bed of dim verdant greens with a basic natively constructed dressing for a meal stuffed with B nutrients for sound methylation and detox pathways.

Fat bombs will control your sweet tooth and give you enough sound fats to continue you until your next meal, and these are particularly fulfilling because they suggest a flavor like cinnamon rolls.

Broccoli is high in cell reinforcements. Salmon is also a top choice for its taste and supplement thickness, however you can choose any wild-got fish based on your personal preference. Serve with a portion of your preferred vegetables cooked in coconut oil, and you have a snappy and simple superfood meal.

Ingredients:

- 1 pound salmon or other fish of choice
- 2 tablespoons crisp lemon juice
- 2 tablespoons ghee
- 4 cloves garlic, finely diced

Preparation:

- Preheat broiler to 400 °F. Combine lemon juice, ghee, and garlic.
- Spot salmon in thwart and pour lemon and ghee blend over the top.
- Wrap salmon with the foil and spot on a preparing sheet.
- Prepare for 15 minutes or until salmon is cooked through.
- If your stove size permits, you can cook your vegetables nearby salmon on a different preparing sheet.

2. Intermediate fasting meal plan.

With this arrangement, you will eat just between the long stretches of 12 p.m. and 6 p.m., for an entire 18 hours of fasting inside a 24-hour time span. You can practice this arrangement during the week's worth of work. If you're not a morning meal person, simply appreciate a couple of cups of home grown tea to begin your day.

Despite the fact that you are skipping breakfast, it's critical to remain hydrated. Try to even drink more water now. You can likewise have home grown tea (most specialists concur that espresso and tea don't break your fast). The catechins in tea have been shown to upgrade the advantages of fasting by assisting with advancing abatement of the appetite hormone, ghrelin, so you can hold until lunch and not feel denied.

Since you've expanded your fasting period an additional four hours, you have to ensure your first meal (around early afternoon) has enough sound fats. A burger in the 8-to-6-window plan will function admirably, and you can include more fats in your dressing or top it with an avocado!

Nuts and seeds make extraordinary snacks that are high-fat and can be eaten around 2:30 p.m. Drenching these heretofore can help kill normally happening catalysts like phytates that can add to stomach related issues. Have the next meal around 5:30 p.m., and simply like in the 8-to-6-window plan, a meal with a wild-got fish or other clean protein source with vegetables is an extraordinary alternative.

First meal, 12 p.m.: Grass-fed burger with avocado

Snack, 2:30 p.m.: Nuts and seeds

Second meal, 5:30 p.m.: Salmon and veggies

3. Propelled: The altered 2-day meal plan.

For this arrangement, eat clean for five days of the week (you can pick whatever days you need). On the other two days, limit your calories to close to 700 every day. Calorie limitation opens a considerable lot of indistinguishable advantages from fasting for a whole day. On your non-fasting days, you'll have to ensure you're getting in solid fats, clean meats, vegetables, and a few natural products, and you can structure your meals anyway best works for you.

On confined days, you can have littler meals or snacks for the duration of the day or have a moderate-size lunch and meal and fast in the first part of the day and after meal. Once more, center around solid fats, clean meats, and produce. Applications can assist you with logging your food and monitor your calorie consumption so you don't go more than 700.

4. Progressed: The 5:2 meal plan.

In this arrangement, you'll eat clean five days of the week, however, you won't eat anything for two non-consecutive days of the week.

For instance, you can fast on Monday and Thursday, however, eat clean meals on different days. Food on these five days will look simply like the rest of the fasting plans—solid fats, clean meat sources, vegetables, and some natural products.

Remember that this arrangement isn't for tenderfoots, and you ought to consistently converse with your primary care physician before beginning any fasting routine, particularly if you are taking drugs or have an ailment. It is prescribed that espresso consumers keep up their morning espresso consumption and that everybody who does a progressed fast remains appropriately hydrated.

- Monday: Fast.
- Tuesday: Eat well; fats, clean meat sources, vegetables, and some natural products.
- Wednesday: Eat well; fats, clean meat sources, vegetables, and some natural products.
- Thursday: Fast.
- Friday: Eat well; fats, clean meat sources,

vegetables, and some natural products.

- Saturday: Eat well; fats, clean meat sources, vegetables, and some natural products.

5. Progressed: Every-other-day plan or substitute day fasting.

Despite the fact that this arrangement is progressed, it's straightforward. Try not to eat anything every other day.

Every other day, eat fats, clean meat sources, vegetables, and some organic products, and afterward on your fasting days, you can consume water, home grown tea, and moderate measures of dark espresso or tea.

- Monday: Eat fats, clean meat sources, vegetables, and some organic products.
- Tuesday: Fast.
- Wednesday: Eat fats, clean meat sources, vegetables, and some natural products.
- Thursday: Fast.
- Friday: Eat fats, clean meat sources, vegetables, and some natural products.
- Saturday: Fast.
- Sunday: Eat fats, clean meat sources,

vegetables, and some natural products.

With this information close by, you should know precisely how to plan meals when beginning an intermittent fasting plan. And keeping in mind that it may appear to be complicated from the outset, when you keep fasting, it will feel natural and fit pretty consistently into your days. Be that as it may, consistently start slow and bit by bit work up to further developed plans.

It's additionally imperative to recollect that you may have some "off" days when intermittent fasting doesn't work for you. Tune in to your body—if you have to eat outside of your average window, it's OK! Simply restart when you're feeling much better.

CHAPTER TEN

FOODS TO ABSOLUTELY AVOID

The most ideal approach to know whether intermittent fasting is suitable for you is to give it a shot and see how it goes.

Would you be able to drink coffee when fasting?

Dark coffee, tea and water are all alright to consume and are not considered to break your fast.

Would you be able to drink bulletproof coffee when you fast?

Shockingly, bulletproof coffee, spread coffees, and coffees with a ton of cream and sugar do break your fast as they contain a considerable amount of calories so try to avoid them.

Would you be able to drink liquor when you intermittent fast?

Drinking liquor would break your fast. So you cannot drink liquor while in your fasting period. You can drink liquor during your eating window.

Notwithstanding, be cautious, make sure to have a meal before consuming liquor and take things moderately. Intermittent fasting may build your affectability to liquor. Drinking a lot of alcohol too fast while intermittent fasting may leave you feeling more awful than anticipated in the first part of the day.

If you're not overweight, would it be a good idea for you to fast?

Fasting isn't just for weight reduction, but it can also prevent ailment and moderate aging.

Broadened fasts might be progressively troublesome or risky for individuals who don't have a lot of muscle versus fat to fuel their fast. Be that as it may, fasting can still be a safe and sound exercise for individuals who are not overweight.

What are the adverse effects of intermittent fasting?

Conceivable negative reactions of intermittent fasting are:

- Yearning
- Migraines
- Stoppage
- Unsteadiness
- Heart Burn
- Muscle Cramps

In fasts that last under 48 hours, as a rule these reactions are not genuine. If manifestations do continue, or if you are anticipating fasting over 48 hours, if it's not too much trouble, consult a specialist.

Would you be able to fast excessively?

No! Fasting again and again or for a really long time can prompt unhealthiness. We suggest you stay with one of the famous timetables recorded above or consult a doctor first.

Will your digestion drop when you fast?

When done correctly, no. A few examinations show that intermittent fasting will actually expand your digestion.

How might I conquer my appetite?

With short fasts, it's all psychological. Yearning will come in waves and will in general deteriorate. Truth be told, in longer fasts, individuals will say their craving leaves after the principal couple of days. Try your best to overlook hunger.

In any case, appetite is often difficult to ignore. If you're experiencing hunger during intermittent fasting, take a stab at drinking a great deal of water or having a coffee. Likewise, focus your brain on an errand and remain occupied to keep your thoughts off eating.

What is the best food to break your intermittent fast? Here are some normal, sound choices used to break a fast:

- MCT Oil
- Nuts
- Bone-stock
- Verdant green lettuces
- Avocado
- Aged foods (yogurt, sauerkraut and so on)

CONCLUSIONS

Combining keto and IF might be viable for certain individuals, but right now, it probably won't be better. The general degree of limitation of doing the two weight control plans together might be overpowering, and on the grounds that each diet has been demonstrated to be successful all alone, there's no convincing motivation to join them, particularly if doing so will affect your capacity to keep up this style of eating as long as possible.

Intermittent Fasting is an extraordinary way to get in shape, renew your cells, and ideally add to your life expectancy. In any case, intermittent fasting isn't for everybody. Finally, wellbeing is tied to eating healthy foods, getting enough rest, diminishing pressure and finding the correct balance.